PRAISE FOR "DON'T LOO[

Jeffrey Stephens: *Master Hypnotist*

"Jon Chase is an amazing hypnotist and a brilliant teacher. ᴀ̄ᴜ ̄
volume is truly a work of art. The straight 'dope' with no nonsense or
wasted material. It lays out all that any person desiring to be a
hypnotist needs to know. It does not cater to the would-be hypnotherapist or psychoanalyst. This book presents the facts and how-to
for those who are desiring to get back to what the founders of this art
used successfully for many years. Induce, test, apply 'remedy', and
bring 'em out feeling better than they went in."

"Having read far more books on hypnosis than I care to count, this
one is among the most useful I have ever seen. I recommend it highly."

DON'T LOOK IN HIS EYES!

how to be a confident original hypnotist

JONATHAN CHASE
"The Dream Pilot"

Don't look in his eyes!
How to be a confident original hypnotist

The right of Jonathan Chase to be identified as the author of this work has been asserted by him in accordance with the UK Copyright, Designs and Patents Act 1988 and all world-wide laws and covenants.

Published in the UK by Academy of Hypnotic Arts Ltd
PO Box 82, Dawlish, Devon. EX7 0WP. UK
www.originalhypnosis.com
First printed edition 2007
Printed and bound in Great Britain
by Antony Rowe

ISBN Number: 978-0-9547098-3-9

With thanks and undying gratitude to everyone
buying this book.
Without you lot people like me
would have nothing to do.

Jonathan Chase

Table of Contents

ACKNOWLEDGEMENTS

I'll head nod here to people like Charles Tebbetts, Jay Ruffley, Robin Colville, Jane Bregazzi, Clare Whiston, Jeff Stephens and all of the other people I have trained or trained with. And I must thank my clients and students and anyone else who has inspired, influenced, led or threatened me into giving you this.

Jon

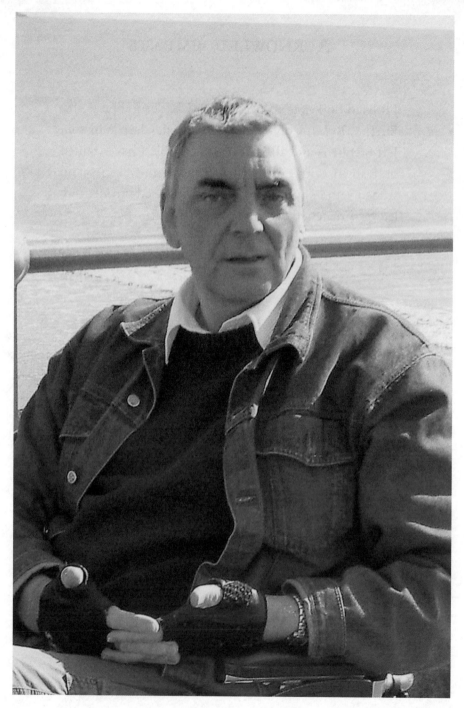

Foreword by Adam Eason

I first encountered Jonathan Chase when I was at a very embryonic stage of my own hypnotherapy career. He was often outspoken, very often he was hilarious and witty, and pretty much all of the time he had lots of information to give that set my curiosity alight. Jon loves the hypnotic arts and this is very evident in his writing and when speaking to him.

Many people shy away from stage hypnosis and some even curl their noses, yet those of us in the know are acutely aware of what it takes to be an outstanding stage hypnotist. As well as being one of the leading figures in this field, Jon then went and wrote one of the best books on that subject (Deeper and deeper) that I have encountered... And I have encountered many.

I was honoured and delighted when Jon asked me to read this latest book and write a foreword. As with many aspects of modern hypnosis, Jon and I have our difference in opinion, perceptions and understanding. You know what though? Jon writes in a style that I find extremely agreeable. Even if I initially disagree with the subject matter, he gets me seeing things differently and is constantly pushing the boundaries of my own understanding and does it so gently and subtly that I hardly realise it is happening, now that is hypnosis.

Despite this book educating and challenging anyone interested in learning more about hypnosis and its therapeutic applications, Jon retains a simple way of writing, even with the most complex of subjects and it makes this book a joy to read.

I particularly enjoy and advocate the fact that this book encourages you to abandon what Jon calls 'scriptnosis.' So many budding hypnotists rattle off scripts and many of the best selling hypnosis books are filled with scripts for you to read to people and bore them to sleep. This book shows you how to be a hypnotist that needs no script. These are the skilled people with the world at their feet.

From one hypnotist to another: Having got hold of a copy of this book, you are going to learn about hypnosis today. You are going to learn what it is all about and you are going to have fun doing so. Read. Enjoy. Read again."

With my very best wishes,

Adam

adam-eason.com

Hello there

I'm sitting at my computer starting this, my second book about hypnosis and what we will be using as the manual for our Personal Development hypnosis training. The first book, Deeper and Deeper the secrets of stage hypnosis, is as I write this out selling all the others on hypnosis on amazon.co.uk. and has been sold on every continent in the world except Antarctica. Which is not bad considering my English teacher emigrated to New Zealand citing me as the reason for her becoming a Hobbit.

But Mrs Oliver was right; I'm not a writer so my apologies in advance for writing the way I speak and for repeating myself on occasion. But then maybe I shouldn't apologise; this is as much a book for your creative subconscious or better still your mind, as it is a book for your logical conscious or brain so plain speaking and imagination exciting will be the order of the day.

I won't use the useless scientific language which has surrounded hypnosis to the point of strangulation, mainly because I don't understand half of it and I've been in the game for a long time and it hasn't seemed to matter. Also because most of this hypnotic language means virtually nothing and is just the lingo of the 'in' crowd. So I hope you will find this very clear, very simple and really accessible

By all means read this book with your Bull Shit radar turned up to maximum and if you get a blip let me know as I have really tried hard not to include any.

Before we begin there is something that I would like to make absolutely clear. It would be impossible in a book this size to tell you everything that there is to know about Hypnosis. So I have included only the stuff that you actually need to know. The rest is window dressing you can add later. And I apologise in advance for the odd ramble, this isn't a technical only manual, you can't have that for an art. That, in my opinion is what hypnosis is, my beautiful art.

Hopefully whether you're a novice or an expert, you'll find something in here that will teach, inform, or maybe something that just excites some thinking. Either way let me know.

Good times and thank you for buying this book.

Smiles

JonC

Original Hypnosis

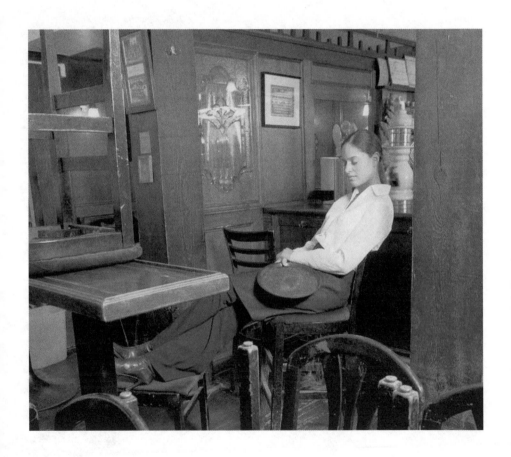

"Everything should be made as simple as possible, but not simpler." Albert Einstein.

When I first started to question the complexity of over a hundred years of **apparent** development of hypnosis, I was accused of arrogance by the majority of leading therapists. How dare I question the work of the great minds that have preceded me and the massive tomes of learned and illustrious work in the fields of psychotherapy and analysis.

Luckily I'm an obstinate cuss and decided to find out why hypnosis works, and if the other stuff like psychotherapy and analysis made it work any better. I figured that if I could get rid of the useless theory which makes things inaccessible to undereducated people like me I'd write a book about it.

I did and here's the book.

If you're the sort of person who believes it takes a computer the size of the average family house and laboratories full of genius geeks to work out something as amazing as E=MC2, you will no doubt find some of this book too simple. What it actually took to describe the universe in such a simple little equation was the pad, pencil, and rather small but massively creative brain of a dyslexic physicist.

You may, even if you buy into a minimalist approach, still think you need more. Many people who attend our learning programmes go off and read thick books full of largely unproven theoretical rubbish. And then most of them, when we get together, admit to coming back to the simply direct, workable, and successful stuff they learned with us. Ultimately the choice is yours; however, I do assure you that everything you need to be a productive hypnotist is

3

here, except of course the practical and personal experience. And it's the experience that makes the difference.

One thing I discovered working out in the real world for all these years is that some things work and some don't. Some are very elegant, sophisticated, and only work partially or at least not acceptably well and are just fun to play with. Some techniques bring almost consistently predictable results and some don't. I'm going to concentrate as much as possible in this book, as I do in my courses, on what works for almost everyone in my experience. And as a hypnotist friend of mine put it, I'll cut to the chase.

One thing is for sure, Hypnosis is one of the most fascinating and illuminating phenomena we can experience. Hypnosis without the overt evangelism of the motivationalist and the complex theorizing of the psychotherapist, is a smart and fast way to simply get better, no matter what better means to you.

Creating problems and issues, or peace and happiness our mind or subconscious uses the same process of communication and inner patterning as it does to create positive and productive behaviours and beliefs. Once we learn how that process can be influenced we can choose which experience we would rather have.

In some quarters, certainly here, Hypnosis is coming of age by returning to its roots and shrugging off the cumbersome and complex additions it has picked up over the last hundred years as more and more artisans learn the real thing.

Not just for smoking and weight reduction, this remarkable and natural state of the human mind can be used to turn desire into reality and to increase the emotional enjoyment and experience of life. Using hitherto ignored or forgotten assets of the greatest creation we know of, ourselves, and to do so at the speed of thought.

It's been said in quantum circles that the mind is the last frontier. If that's true then hypnosis is the Starship Enterprise and hypnotists are its crew. Let's hope that we can see more use of this wonderful state of mind for play, such as increasing the enjoyment of sex, for human evolution in helping to expand and develop psychic abilities, and in education where we could teach faster and create potentially happier people.

There's an old saying that '*happiness is a journey not a destination.*' I'll go with that, and add that no one said we have to crawl. To that end this is a book about rapid approaches and how you can learn at speed. Actually that's cheating because all we need to do is tell you how to use what you already know and do but don't notice.

Hypnosis is big and it is clever – when done deliberately. Real hypnosis is clever but isn't rocket science, it isn't science at all, it's art, which means anyone can do it regardless of education or academic achievement.

I'm going to give you understanding of something I've observed working every day and for the whole of my life, but for only a few decades with understanding. If you are expecting loads of history and quotes from other people's books you'll be disappointed, there are too few managed woodlands to repeat what's gone before, buy their books.

Obviously this book leans towards becoming a **professional** hypnotist, and so it more than likely will have bits in it that not everybody needs to know. But stick with it because I know that you'll find something in here for you.

In this book hypnosis is precisely that, just hypnosis. Real hypnosis. It has been called Ultradepth and Ultraheight, Somnambulism, the Esdaile state, Mesmerism, NLP and lots of other stuff. At the end of the day it's all just hypnosis.

Everything here has been used, examined, performed or played with for real. I know everything in here works because I've done it or seen it happen. And I know it can work for you because I have seen it happen for others just like you in our learning programmes, hundreds of times.

Naturally there are also some snippets of my own philosophy, but this is my book.

Finally I've lost count of the number of times I've been asked what the difference is between a hypnotherapist and a hypnotist. In my book the difference becomes apparent when you ask the question.

A hypnotherapist will undoubtedly suggest that you make an appointment, then spend the next fifteen minutes explaining why it may not work and how you can't be forced to do something…

A hypnotist, certainly one trained by me, will tell you to sit down or stand just so and within seconds you'll know what the difference is.

Oh yes and I know you can be a hypnotist because you already are, **you** just don't know it yet.

Hypnotic History

Now most books I have ever read on hypnosis begin with a mention of the art's history, and now we've mentioned it we can move on.

I'm working on the understanding that when you buy a computer you don't need to know who invented it, improved it or made it worse to enable you to use it. On the previous page I've mentioned some names which you should look up on the internet or your library if you are a history buff.

It is my experience that history often confuses and misinterprets things and as I've said this really is a simple book written for those who want to know what works in practice today, and how to use that.

In my experience those people who don't actually use Hypnosis, but use some light relaxation along with visualisation, are the ones who talk most of the people like James Braid, whilst totally ignoring the deep state of hypnosis he and our other forefathers used.

Originally hypnotism was about suggestion and inducing a state to facilitate the acceptance of suggestion. Then, due to a lack of understanding by observers, it came to be associated with sleep and relaxation which the original hypnosis most certainly wasn't.

Mesmer, Braid, Esdaile, Charcot, Elman, Erickson. These giants of hypnosis share one little known secret, not one of them used relaxation. They were all suggestion hypnotists.

They used eye fixation on lights and shiny objects. They induced by making passes, that's waving your hands in a downward motion, in front of people. They used what I call 'Wide awake' hypnosis – non trance states.

And they did all of this with a success rate that beggars belief when put up against so-called cutting edge methods.

Among these pages you will get an insight to these methods. But I'm not going to bore you with a life story of all of these guys after all; you don't need to know all about the Roman Empire to make a pizza taste good.

The Conscious, Unconscious, and ∫ubconscious

I know I'm not alone in this, and there are plenty more people just as confused and befuddled by the almost ballistic use of the above words as I am.

Hopefully to aid clarity in this book, I've decided to use what I consider to be the most accurate understanding, and the simplest one, of what these things are.

Conscious: The Brain

The conscious matures. It grows up. It is the seat of logic and of reason, both of which are noticeably absent from children under the age of nine or so years. This is not an absolute and it can differ immensely from individual to individual. But there is no doubt in my mind that we are not born with logic.

In some individuals, and according to most female authors on the subject 'some individuals' includes all males, such maturity never happens and they never 'grow up' or develop logical thinking. But for the sake of not wanting to write that particular book, let's just agree that the majority do and that happens at around nine years and six months old.

The brain is an organic computer and it differs from other computers we use only because it is aware of itself as an entity. We know this because it uses the term 'I' a lot. It understands that the world it inhabits is a complex and convoluted place in which the reality it shares with other similar beings is one of subtle interplay and cooperation, of judgment and opinion, of logic and reason. It's wrong but . . .

All of these realisations and skills appear to increase in application if not efficiency over a period with the human state usually known as childhood. The older we get the better we get at reasoning.

As logic and reasoning become better with age I think that conscious is therefore the result of the physical programming of our organic computer and I will therefore be using the words brain and conscious to mean the same thing.

Unconscious: Nothing

My understanding of the word unconscious is that of being comatose. Maybe my past in nursing has coloured my opinion on this word but in my experience unconscious folk tend to lie around and not do a lot.

How this word came to be connected with the thought process that occurs during hypnosis is beyond my understanding. Okay, hypnosis doesn't involve the conscious too much but we do know that the conscious is active to the degree that we can use language to have a conversation with a hypnotised person so they are not entirely unconscious.

I have seen a lot of unconscious people. They are terrible conversationalists. I do understand that we've been saddled with this inaccurate term because it could vaguely explain involuntary behaviour, such as blood circulation and balance which to my way of thinking are way more mechanical than people realise and don't need thought to work at all. It makes no sense using unconscious to explain emotive behaviour.

So, for the purpose of this book I'm going to take the approach that I think is most useful to apply to this word in hypnotic terms, I'm going to ignore it altogether.

ſubconscious: The Mind

The prefix 'sub' in this context has become to be understood as being below or beneath. Maybe that's what led to phrases such as 'deeper and deeper' and 'levels' of trance.

The question must be - below or beneath what?

I rather think that the 'sub' in subconscious was applied by the founders of psychology to mean subordinate. One of the hardest things to get people to admit to is always the fact that they are not in control. Or rather that their conscious mind is not the dominant and controlling part of their mental process. Psychoanalysis doesn't admit this at all. In fact much of its clinical application relies on making the conscious mind aware of past traumatising events in the presumption that the dominant conscious can then correct any behaviour that resulted from that experience. This is rubbish. The vast majority of clients I've had knew exactly when and where their problems started and were still totally unable to do anything about them.

I think Einstein was right when he said,
"The intuitive mind is a sacred gift and the rational mind is a faithful servant. We have created a society that honours the servant and has forgotten the gift."

The conscious brain is the servant.

I fail to see how anyone could miss this. No matter what you think consciously or even want to do consciously if there is not agreement from your Mind it will not happen. You may want to stop smoking, over-eating, biting your nails, to stop being stressed all of the time at the logical level. But unless this is emotively supported you will not change your behaviour.

The Mind is therefore quite simply, and absolutely without question, the strongest and most governing part of our mental make-up. It is certainly not **sub** anything.

It is the seat of your desires, your hopes, and your fears. It is your best friend and yes, at times, your worst enemy. It's the place where you really live. Your mind is the centre of your emotions and your behaviours, your reality and your beliefs. Maybe it's the only part of you that is real, maybe not.

So for the purposes of this book

BRAIN = CONSCIOUS
AND
MIND = SUBCONSCIOUS

What is Hypnosis?

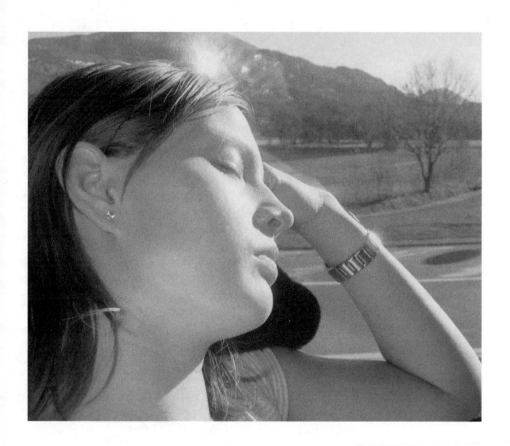

On the Academy of Hypnotic Arts' website we describe hypnosis thus: Hypnosis is the art of producing changes in our mental patterning by the use of a sometimes deliberate act of communication and influence of the human emotional and belief patterning system, achieved by reducing and / or redirecting the attention of the logical conscious process so that the mind [subconscious] becomes directly contactable.

And *that* really is that, although 'hypnosis' also describes the art itself.

Hypnosis isn't relaxation, sleep, or any derivative. For that reason, what most people think of as hypnotic or hypnotherapy is usually what many hypnotists have come to refer to as relaxotherapy. That is, relaxation with some psychotherapy thrown in.

I'm not knocking this way of working. In many cases this is very productive and sometimes even beneficial to the client, and this book shouldn't put you off using such an approach as a hypnotist. Sometimes using relaxation is a good way of inducing those people who need to have it. It is important however that you understand that in the majority of cases hypnotherapy just using relaxation without testing or giving suggestions is not really hypnosis.

Probably the best example most people know of hypnosis is that seen on stage. There is nothing wrong with that because without the showmanship and the target of entertaining an audience it is this state that the earliest hypnotists used and to which the word refers. So stage hypnosis is **real** hypnosis.

The prefix 'stage' describes the environment and the target [entertainment] rather than the act or the state. And most importantly this is the model of hypnosis which is deeply embedded in the zeitgeist or shared conscious of any society with a television or a cinema. It is what people expect.

Hypnosis is a specific state of mind, a state which is induced – that is caused by someone or something else – and one in which the unquestioning and most powerful part of our mind accepts without reserve any reality imposed upon it.

When hypnotised we expect to experience the unquestioning acceptance of suggestion, regardless of how illogical or strange those may be, along with the capability to hallucinate both positively and negatively at the drop of a suggestion, and to have full focus on the hypnotist.

It is the hypnotist who is then in control and in charge, although no hypnotist can **force** anyone to do anything, this isn't necessary. The concept of force is wrong; direction and instruction and even persuasion and manipulation are more accurate terms.

When the communication and focus of the belief system is entirely directed at the hypnotist, he/she can persuade, influence and cajole in a very profound and lasting way.

A hypnotist can and does affect the mind in the same way as a traumatic or deeply emotional event can. If that doesn't happen then what you have is a chat or counselling, you certainly don't have hypnosis.

For that reason professional hypnosis for remedial reasons carries with its practice a good deal of responsibility and if you play with any of the practical aspects of this book know that you are taking on that responsibility.

How Does Hypnosis Work?

Have you ever watched a parent yell at a child in such a way that the child, who is about as open to suggestion as you can be in your whole life, especially before the age of nine, takes that suggestion and becomes 'programmed' or patterned to do or not do something?

In this instance we see emotive state and directive suggestion when the kid is about to grab the boiling pan and play Vesuvius with his head. The parent yells **"NO!"** and scares the kid nearly to death. Because of the fear induced hyper–emotional state – and the following hugs and kisses and tears and nappy change – the subconscious mind is dominant and the suggestion bypasses the conscious. In most cases, the child is hypnotised and the pattern established never to scald himself.

That is hypnosis. At least it is the same process—the delivery and acceptance of a suggestion that causes a change in the internal patterns that govern behavior or belief while the emotive and controlling part of us is open and totally dominant.

Now let's go and look at the couple across the street to see how this form of 'natural' hypnosis works just as well for adults.

They are having a row and he's just told her that she is fat, frosty, and bloody boring.

She is emotive and not being too logical. In fact for the moment her conscious logical brain is taking a back seat and the mind is out there handling the hurt and throwing back some dirt of its own. At that point his suggestions go right in there and if accepted become patterns. Moreover, unless she is lucky enough to have the opposite happen from some other non-aware hypnotist or she visits a good knowing one, she could react to that suggestion and have a lot of trouble with relationships from here on in, if she has them at all.

The art of hypnosis is on display and in use constantly all around us and all the time. The shame is we do not know it and so don't use it fruitfully all of the time. Just imagine when consoling someone in a traumatic emotive state that your suggestions of 'time being a great healer' are accepted and as a result, that person suffers their grief for much longer than was needed. A properly formulated and delivered suggestion at this point such as, "From tomorrow things will begin to be better" could have the effect of shortening the length of suffering.

It isn't a superhuman gift or anything magical – well not in the Merlin sense anyway. It may appear to be a miracle although it is not miraculous. It's the art of using what we do all the time and doing it deliberately and with intent.

So hypnosis works when a suggestion by-passes our conscious logic and becomes accepted by our mind as fact.

It is important to know that the mind does not reason, it just chooses, and acceptance of suggestion happens or it doesn't.

The brain is logical, it can tell the difference between outside reality and make-believe and construction, whereas the mind perceives reality entirely from the patterns it holds and has no idea of any difference between reality and fantasy. It can accept suggestions simply because it feels like it or because that suggestion matches one already accepted as reality.

If the idea of patterns is confusing, think of it like this. To remember something, your mind creates a pattern of connections in your brain and body and for all we know in other places and dimensions as well. It is these patterns or models we access when we have to decide what to do about, or with, something happening in our lives.

Some of these are hard-wired instincts. Throw a brick at someone's head and providing you throw it from the front or shout "duck", they will move out of the way. [Don't try this at home].
We call these hard-wired patterns Instincts and there are not too many of them.

Eat something, drink something, see a member of the opposite gender and sh… Well you get the idea.

Have a look at a group of human infants; you'll see they are the same in beliefs, responses, wants, needs. Their innate desires regardless of sex, race, creed or lack of McDonald's will be the same.

All the other stuff is taught to us. Learnt makes it sound like logical and sensible. And although these are involved in the mind of the teacher, for the student they don't appear until much later than the first four or five years, the time when we do most of our learning.

We know that if we put a cross-section of kids in a compound somewhere and gave them all the same input that we would come out with people with much the same belief and response systems, the same patterns.

You don't have to look much further than Northern Ireland, Palestine, or even the UK to see that in action.

We do put kids in these boxes and it's here where most lay hypnosis takes place. We call these boxes schools, churches and even societies.

That's hypnosis without the official label. With the official label, it's fair to say that hypnosis is direct communication with the dominant mind in such a way that such communication creates patterns that permanently alter behaviour and belief.

When we say that hypnosis is communication in which we talk directly to the mind, I can't stress enough the fact that communication is not just language. If it were then we'd have no advertisements with scantily dressed young people seductively lounging in boats and erotically slurping in the latest chocolate bar TV ad, and the world would be a far sadder place in my opinion.

Communication takes many forms and the guess seems to be that only ten percent of this is language. This is a guess of course, and one in which so many people believe now it's grown some truth. Communication both external and internal happens all the time and I've never figured out how you can manage to grade it or break it up into percentages but science is a wonderful thing and can do anything it wants to really.

Therefore, a predominant part of hypnosis is the acceptance of suggestion using direct communication with the mind; and as with any communication, we have to understand that suggestion doesn't have to be words.

It can just as easily be visual as in the outward manifestation of emotion, a laugh or a tear. It can be kinetic such as a caress or a blow. It can be auditory as in scream or a snippet of music or taste or smell or any experience.

The way we walk and move communicates, as does every twitch, shake or smile. In fact, language, either as you are now using it to read this internally to yourself, or if you are listening to it, is only the tool of the logical conscious brain.

The rest of you, the mind, is listening to everything else. The choice of font, the feel of the paper, the smell of the ink, the room temperature, the tone of voice, yours or mine. Moreover, it is really listening.

I always tell attendees on our learning programmes to remember this vital fact, that when you become a hypnotist and are accepted as such by the people you're working with, then everything you say, do, or even think will become a suggestion.

Because everything you think, say, or do will be received as communication by the mind of the hypnotee.

What Does Hypnosis Feel Like?

When you are hypnotised it feels like green.

Really good green.

Like really smooth and warm and silky green.

Unless it feels blue of course.

I've never yet met anyone who hasn't at some point wondered what hypnosis will feel like. And I've never yet been able to tell them. My stock reply is, "Just come here and tell me what it felt like in a minute."

One thing for absolute certain is - it feels like HYPNOSIS! - and everyone who has been there **knows** it.

Most "hypnosis" in the marketplace actually isn't.

I shudder every time I read the old myth on the internet "You will not be out of 'control', and at any time you wish you will be able to end the session and just walk away". If you are a little relaxed and you can stand up and just walk away then you are not hypnotised. This is just relaxation. I don't go for this light level of hypnosis stuff and when you read the early books of the guys who operated on thousands of people, they didn't either.

I really do believe that these light levels and the mass acceptance of hypnosis being a state in which you remain 'in control', or can just get up and walk away from, was originally nothing more than an excuse for failure or a therapist's cop out. I don't know where this rubbish comes from but when you consider that one of the original hypnotists, James Braid, was a surgeon who performed eye operations using hypnosis as the only anaesthetic. It would have been unfortunate and very messy if somebody had just got up and walked away in the middle of the procedure.

When I'm hypnotised I don't 'feel' anything much. At least if I do I'm not aware of it in any cognitive sense. I couldn't care less where or even when I am, and I'm totally focused on nothing I can logically get a hold of.

If I can notice anything at all then it feels like it isn't me and I'm a million miles away watching somebody else be hypnotised.

When I come out I will definitely be aware of what happened if the hypnotist has told me I will, otherwise it's hit and miss and I'll usually give up trying to recall because it doesn't seem important.

I usually feel a little spaced out and have no idea how long I've been in there. I often feel a warm glow and refreshed because that's how my hypnotist brings me back from where ever it is she's taken me. [My partner Jane Bregazzi being my hypnotist usually].

That's how I feel. And strangely enough, it's how most of the people I have hypnotised describe that thing as well.

Almost always there is partial or complete amnesia. This is spontaneous although if you don't want this to happen it's easily turned round by just telling them they will remember everything.

There is always temporal distortion because time is a conscious logical thing which the mind happily ignores.

How the hypnotees are going to feel I've no idea. But I do know that if they decide they've had enough and just walk away then they are not hypnotised.

I am aware that there are those who say they tell people this lie in the same way as one would lie to a child to protect it from something –
"Don't sit too close to the TV your eyes will go square!"
"Stop throwing that ball, you'll have someone's eye out!"
"Your face will stick like that when the wind changes!"

I'd like to think that it was a useful 'protection' for people I talk to about hypnosis but it isn't. I'd like to think it was even just a simple lie to persuade the hypnotee to go along with the hypnosis, such as when your doctor tells you this is only going to be a sharp scratch when they are forcing a piece of tubular steel the size of an Alaskan oil pipeline into your butt.

The actuality is that most hypnotists – certainly therapists – actually believe this is true. And this is a great shame because it does often mean that they never see hypnosis, and miss witnessing the amazingly rapid - and often instant - changes in personality their clients are capable of.

From the hypnotists' point of view the state of hypnosis is characterised by one common factor in all cases, **the unquestioning acceptance of suggestions.**

Is Hypnosis Harmful?

The state of hypnosis itself and its accompanying phenomena are not harmful. In fact most people find that just being hypnotised is very restorative and enlightening. I've had people return to me regularly just to experience the state.

One business man used to come along, get "zapped", and I'd go make a cup of tea for myself while he got what he called his "battery recharge".

I was told at one of the many courses and seminars I've attended over the years that giving regular hypnosis experiences without any actual therapy was wrong, probably immoral, and would lead to the client becoming dependant on the hypnotist. However in this – my book – there is nothing wrong with that. People visit massage parlours of the reputable and other kind on a regular basis, and have their cars serviced once a year, are dependant on their baker, doctor, tobacconist. So why not have a regular mind massage? I don't think being depended on is dangerous.

The fact is that hypnosis is a mood and nothing more.

So the state of hypnosis isn't dangerous in itself, however what you do within the state as a hypnotist can be, and has been, detrimental to people.

I shudder when I read that hypnosis is 'harmless' because you won't do anything harmful or inappropriate to yourself and therefore would never accept a suggestion likely to cause harm. Apparently this isn't possible because you have a safety valve which stops anything inappropriate becoming a belief or behaviour.

If that is true then why then do people who are regularly behaving in an inappropriate or unproductive way, those who because they were told whilst in an emotive state that they were useless and have spent the next twenty years being just that, seek out hypnosis? They must have accepted the suggestion that caused this somewhere.

The fact is that hypnosis is just as dangerous as any other human interchange, whether that be professional or not. And I always think it's a bit of an insult to people's intelligence to tell them that they can't be harmed by incompetence.

Not accepting this possibility and its attending responsibility when learning how to easily affect the way others think is like being a guy with a loaded gun who believes that if he doesn't pull the trigger the beast is safe so he doesn't bother to put on the safety catch. The majority of gun shot wounds and deaths are in fact accidental and not recognising the potential danger is what causes these accidents.

One fact of hypnosis is that if you cannot implant a phobia you cannot remove one. And that is what the hypnotist does; removes the pattern causing the unproductive, inappropriate, and limiting behaviour, and hopefully instills a more productive way of reacting to things.

To do this we use exactly the same mental process to remove the patterned behaviour as was used to install it.

A good metaphor to use when asked this question is, "Is a scalpel dangerous in the hands of a surgeon? Hopefully no, because they recognize and understand what it is they are holding and take responsibility for its use. Hypnosis is no different."

An obvious danger we often get asked about is can you get stuck in hypnosis, and the answer is a firm no. A rubber band, when it's stretched taut, doesn't stay stretched when you let go. Your mind works in a similar fashion; when the hypnotist or conditions let go, it springs back to its usual state of attention. Sooner or later.

Even so, as with any human endeavour the responsibility and recognition of the capabilities of the methods we are using should be recognised.

Remember, if you can harm when you're not a **deliberate** hypnotist, and you give a suggestion which stays with someone their whole life, you most certainly can do harm when you are a deliberate hypnotist. The only way to ensure that you don't do this is to accept that you can.

I know, you've read that a hypnotist can't make you do anything that goes against your will. That's fine, except for the fact that your will is part of your conscious; and lets face it, that's pants at doing much for us. If will was able to resolve things then we'd all be thinking perfectly and hypnosis wouldn't be a profession in any other way than as a form of entertainment. Interestingly, 'will' is easy to overcome; your mind does it all the time.

We can 'will' not smoking, overeating, jumping out of skins at the sight of a crane fly or not making every relationship become the same disaster as all the others, and well…

So much for will.

The thing is hypnosis doesn't need to force against the will, it just circumvents it, or simply changes it because your will is a construct

31

of your physical logical brain, and in hypnosis it doesn't much matter what that's doing.

Conscious will is based on what the brain perceives as the required action for social acceptability and the mind couldn't care less about that.

When did you last see a drunk or a football hooligan consciously aware of being socially unacceptable? Remove the logic of social responsibility and you remove the will.

If you're reading this book out of interest and are considering going to a hypnotist I do hope this section doesn't put you off. Hopefully it may get you to ask the question in the title with a little more comprehension and understanding of the answer.

It should be said that if the unbending belief of the hypnotist is that no harm can happen then this does reduce the chances. Judge whether or not you work with the person by the clarity of their answers to your questions.

False Memory Syndrome

There is a lot of it about apparently. A search on Google brought about 880,000 pages. This is where someone doing analysis is responsible for creating or suggesting or even just encouraging a memory of an experience which did not happen.

This could be the 'memory' of an abuse which changes the relationship between a person and their parents. It could lead to worse problems than you started with.

The thing is that all memory is partially the realty of the event and partially false. And as the one thing hypnosis does best is to increase the capability of imagination and creativity I wouldn't personally trust a thing that came from a hypnotised mind and would treat this as what it is. A subjective metaphorical creation.

And as with all other hypnotic dangers this is simple to avoid. Don't analyze. There is no 100% believable research that proves conclusively that going back to a memory and becoming consciously aware of why you started a particular behaviour sorts anything. In fact in hypnosis you could just tell someone you did that and that their problem is sorted and guess what? It will be.

However not to worry the Diagnostic and Statistical Manual of Mental Disorders discredits false memory syndrome as – well – false, and so you should be okay.

Is Hypnosis A Natural Phenomenon?

Yes, it is a natural phenomenon, and not at all like the usual explanations you're likely to read elsewhere.

Hypnosis happens 'naturally' when we are in a state where logic goes flying through the window, and when our conscious - and often our conscience - are no longer dominant.

These are the times when our normal focus shifts and we stop thinking and just act. Those times when afterwards you find yourself thinking 'Why did I say that?' and 'What the hell was I thinking of?'

At these times the mind is dominant. By dominant I mean that it is the part of our mental process which is receiving input from the outside world and acting on that almost exclusively.

It's fair to say that hypnosis also occurs naturally from birth until the physical brain and its attendant conscious thought process mature.

For the first five years or so we are almost constantly hypnotically open. For that reason you learn more in the first five years of life than you do in the next twenty. That state of openness continues to a lesser degree up to about the age of nine when the physical brain reaches maturity and the full-blown conscious kicks in and takes over 'growing up'. It's for that reason when you do most things with people in hypnosis it helps to think that you will deal with a bright nine-year-old child because the mind doesn't get much past that state of emotional dominance.

Incidents of naturally occurring hypnosis happen when we are highly emotive; scared, angry, or even head over heels in love or lust. These are times when our mind is dominant and can be influenced directly. These are the times when inappropriate patterns are formed such as phobias and unfortunate habits, inappropriate and unproductive beliefs. It is also when we develop all the good stuff like social compliance and kindness, so it isn't all bad.

A lot of established thinking associates hypnosis with day-dreaming or being engrossed in something. Comparing day- dreaming or dissociation, or the lack of recall we experience when driving a familiar route to hypnosis, or when becoming immersed in a book or TV show, is like comparing my back yard with a smattering of snow in February to the Antarctic.

They may look similar but…

Let's just clarify something here before we go further because I'm sick and tired of reading these things when even the slightest experimentation and applied thought just blow them away.

Hypnosis has nothing to do with daydreaming or getting lost in a book. It may look similar, admittedly. However, I have yet to meet the person, myself included, who can successfully implant a positive or negative hallucination in someone who is daydreaming.

Yes, their focus is diverted but internally. With hypnosis there is always external focus – on the hypnotist – otherwise the damn thing wouldn't work. Try giving a suggestion to someone engrossed reading a book and you'll just annoy them, if they notice you at all, and that anger is again of course internal focus.

The other common misapprehension is that you enter hypnosis when you are driving or doing something repetitive, this is just rubbish. You don't remember your familiar journey to work every day unless something remarkable happens because if you consciously remembered everything you would go do-lally flip. Sorry, insane.

If you really think about it, you can always remember. This is just not paying attention to the familiar. It isn't a state where you aren't thinking. Actually what you are usually doing is rehearsing the meeting you are heading to, talking to people in the car, listening to the radio. Just because you don't remember actually driving doesn't make it a hypnotic state. You don't remember sleeping or breathing and these aren't particularly hypnotic either.

Again, try giving someone a suggestion while they are driving and it won't take, unless they are extremely emotional and the mind is dominant. If this isn't the case mostly they will ask you what the hell you are going on about because they are fully conscious and absolutely unhypnotised in every way.

Of course, a good hypnotist can instill suggestions almost anywhere and any time, but they need to create the state first. You'll learn this later, but not when the focus of attention is entirely centered on self. It has to be centered on the hypnotist.

When asked, the daydreamer knows exactly what the daydream was about and knew he was participating in it, and when prodded, the driver will remember the drive. The recall is fragmentary because there is simply no *need* to remember, not because he can't.

As you'll find out with hypnosis this isn't the case.

Who Are The Hypnotists?

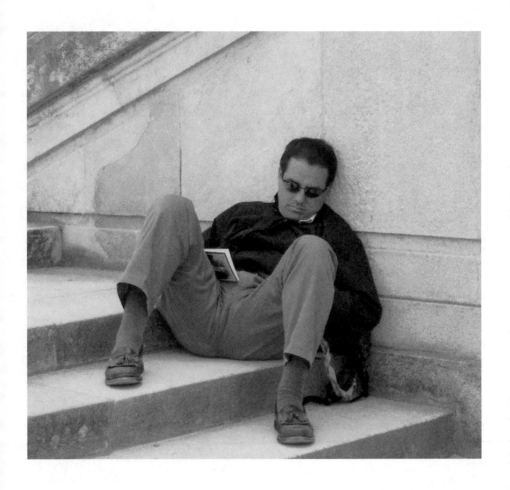

A hypnotist invokes and manages the creative state of hypnotic focus facilitating rapid and permanent change in our emotional patterning when working remedially, or creates a new but temporary reality when working for fun.

The thing is that if you take away the management side of it then everyone uses Hypnosis and everyone becomes a Hypnotic subject at some time in their life. Parents, teachers and significant others all instill belief and behaviour patterns either by direct communication with the mind or by experience, but always bypassing the critical logical brain and delivering suggestion direct to the mind. Everyone learns using this process.

Personally I think that is how learning by repetition works. If you repeat something often enough, sooner or later you will say it at a time when the mind is dominant and natural hypnosis occurs. Or if you say it in such a way that you *create* that emotive and hypnotic state. When that happens the suggestion is accepted and the learning is done. That explains why with some kids it doesn't matter how much you repeat something, it never goes in. For some reason their mind is never excited emotionally to the point where it becomes dominant. That is, they never become hypnotised, at least not in the class.

Now some people have developed their expertise and enhanced their understanding of such communication skills to a point where they can **deliberately** and **systematically** channel their intent and use suggestions to produce a specific state of mind and the resulting effects in other human beings to change and re-pattern the internal reality of another. These people are the Hypnotists.

The better hypnotists I know - better being subjective of course - do seem to share certain traits the most obvious of which is always their confidence. The real hypnotists always have an unbending knowledge that they can 'put anyone under'. They don't believe this, it goes beyond belief. They just know it. Just as you know you will still be you tomorrow. They generally ooze self belief from every pore.

There is also an unbending faith and belief system which gives rise to a passionate conviction in whatever it is they do.

Not all the best hypnotists are Hypnotists by profession of course, but strangely most people understand what it is they do whether they wear the label or not. How many times have you been mesmerised by a passionate speaker, entranced by a fervent teacher or parent, beguiled by a fanatical friend or spellbound by an appealing child?

Even the descriptive language we use shows our deep understanding of what, where, and with whom hypnosis belongs. And because at some time, whether you remember it or not, you will have done one of the above, then it is without doubt safe to say this…

The answer to the question "Who are the hypnotists?" is…

You are.

You just may not know it yet.

Who can be hypnotised?

If you accept that hypnosis is the delivery and acceptance of suggestion then the answer is of course – everyone. However if you are asking who can be induced to enter a trance state which displays certain phenomena then the answer is – everyone who can freely imagine and express that creativity in such a way that can be understood by others.

Autistic people can in my opinion be hypnotised, we may not be able to understand the observable state.

Downs syndrome people are the other end of the spectrum and show the effects of the hypnotic state way more easily than the bulk of so called normal people.

There's a line of thought that some people make better hypnotic 'subjects' than others. I think this is not quite the case. Some people can look and act *more* hypnotised than others and I think this is because some people are better at following the suggestions and directions of the hypnotist than others.

The thing is that after you have been hypnotised a few times you do get more adept at entering the state of mind and displaying the expected behaviour the operator is looking for. Not because you are better hypnotized, but because you are better at *being* hypnotised.

The other event that may be responsible for this line of thought is the obvious one, that sometimes the methods of the hypnotist in question are not doing the job.

Now as hypnotists go I am the best. Just as every other hypnotist is. This isn't arrogance, it is necessary confidence.

However sometimes I do not work firing all guns. Sometimes, although very rarely, I am not quite perfect and I screw up. Sometimes my fantastic and encyclopaedic knowledge lets me down and whatever it takes to hypnotise the person in front of me just doesn't manifest.

Sometimes I fail. About 1 or 2 percent. This is not indicative of the level of resistance from the hypnotee, nor is it showing how good, bad or indifferent they are to hypnosis. What it is showing is that **I** am fallible. I know that's hard to take in but for a moment just try.

I have always said on my courses,
"I know that everyone can be hypnotised, and I also know that I may not be able to hypnotise everyone."

And I also know that I will get someone writing to me telling me that it's that knowing that stops me hypnotising everyone.

Fair enough. I guess I'll settle for just being outstanding as perfect isn't what I aim for anyway.

ſelf ſuggestion

The question is "Can I 'hypnotise' myself?"

No. At least not in the same way or as intensely as a hypnotist can induce things. There is school of thought that all hypnosis is self hypnosis because the hypnotised person has to allow this to happen. That's pants.

If that's true then all education is self education. All government is self government and all surgery is self surgery and that truly only happens in films.

The thing is, hypnosis results in immediate response and I have rarely seen that in self hypnosis. Unless of course the person involved has been hypnotising themselves to get an instant response over some time. That is not hypnosis as we are understanding the thing here – the state and practice as it was used originally – rather that is the result of self suggestion which is not the same thing at all. Repetition of self suggestion can and does work over time. Relaxing deliberately is nice, but this is not the same as hypnosis.

Hypnosis – and we are talking here about the observed and reported state for which the word was actually invented - requires that suggestions work. It also requires that there be a hypnotist or an hypnotising event which is outside of the hypnotised person. There is no such thing in reality as self hypnosis, and that the focus is on that hypnotist and not on self.

Let's look at that in more depth.

As hypnosis requires your conscious to be by-passed, turned off, ignored, suppressed and your subconscious to become dominant, then it should be obvious that this is not happening if **you** are directing your mind using your conscious. It is possible with practice to actually turn your conscious mind off so that the mind is just left to its own devices without any direction; that is meditation, which isn't hypnosis either.

Listening to recordings whether made by yourself or bought commercially is also not self hypnosis, the hypnotist is directing things, not your conscious. And the chance of initiating a true hypnotic state is very rare. Although this style of delivering suggestion can and does work, it just isn't hypnosis. It's self suggestion.

Obviously self suggestion is very important in our lives. We give ourselves suggestions constantly. But there is a problem with this; most of the suggestions we give ourselves are simply confirmation of unwanted behaviour or beliefs and not a replacement or adjustment of these.

"I don't know why I bother. I'm crap at this!" is a prime example of the suggestions that most people give themselves all of the time.

One of the first truly useful self suggestions invented in the late 1800's by Emile Coue was "Every day in every way I am getting better and better." Sadly this has become terribly clichéd and even though it works just as well as the bad stuff we tell ourselves all the time it is now largely ignored.

Starring at candles, spots on walls or just going into an imaginary scenario floating down rivers et al is not hypnosis. Meditation, yes, hypnosis, no. Hypnosis requires communication directly with the mind without conscious intervention. Only someone else can do that.

We can't hypnotise ourselves, so can we get close to bypassing the conscious? Yes – we can overload it.

Try this – say Banana to yourself until it makes absolutely no sense. Until the word becomes just a sound.

At this point the conscious stops paying attention and the mind takes over. Something is repeating the sound and running the patterns that go with that sound, but it isn't the conscious brain so it must be the mind. Now you are giving yourself a suggestion in as close a manner to actual hypnosis as you are ever likely to get on your own.

The reason this is so similar to hypnosis is because you just bypassed your conscious mind. Your conscious deals with logic. It doesn't do a very good job of fantasy or anything else that doesn't make sense like behaviours and beliefs. We know this from the times where we are consciously totally dominated and we look at a piece of art and it makes no sense to our logic.

However when we are dominated by our mind not our brain, we can take the most obscure and senseless artefacts and make a complete and utter 'artistic' sense of them, we can accept them into our inner reality.

Anything that targets our mind rather than our brain can be considered to be a suggestion, or a symbol. In that case anything bearing the labels of art or fantasy is also hypnotic and that's another way of bypassing the conscious.

When making suggestions to yourself you should be artistic. In other words don't be logical, be as fantastic and as creative as possible. As illogical as possible. You must bypass your conscious brain and get your mind working and dominant. Remember the times we said when this happens naturally, when you're experiencing emotional overload.

The trick here is to be more concerned about how you're feeling than it is about what you are saying. So when using self suggestion always imagine how it would feel to achieve whatever it is you are aiming at.

From here it is an easy step to get your imagination working. Let's give you a quick example.

Say you want to increase your recall (people don't have bad memories - they have inefficient recall). Just think how it would feel to be in a situation where your recall of facts and figures is astounding everyone around you - including you.

Get a handle on the emotions you're feeling and don't worry if these include pride, achievement, a little bit of self-satisfaction. There's absolutely nothing wrong with these so any feelings of worrying about other people saying you're arrogant squish them. Concentrate on what makes you feel good not bad.

Now use whatever phrase comes to mind that seems to be right for how you are feeling. When I do this for recall I get the feeling that 'full', is the phrase I should use.

Now I can enter a suggestion by repeating 'full' over and over and over, until it becomes virtually a mantra, until it makes no **sense**.

In this way I am anchoring the phrase 'full' to feeling quite pleased with myself, which is an emotional state that tends to happen to us rather than being instigated by us.

After I've done this a few times the suggestion becomes automatic the moment I think about remembering something. In other words it becomes auto-suggestion. At that point I don't even need to do anything anymore, which is what we always try and achieve with hypnosis. So I guess it's okay to call that self hypnosis, even though self hypnosis doesn't exist.

I'll just mention CHiNOSIS™ here. Although it is not designed to be in anyway self hypnosis we developed this hypnotic technique to be self administered. It doesn't use suggestion, it incorporates Hypnotic Symbolism and self applied acupressure and is capable of doing everything self hypnosis claims to be able to do without the stress of trying to get into a trance state.

You can get more details from www.chinosis.com for Chinosis. And you will find a little booklet for free detailing self suggestion on the web site www.originalhypnosis.com called "Are you hypnotised? and what to do about it"

What Can Hypnosis Be Used For?

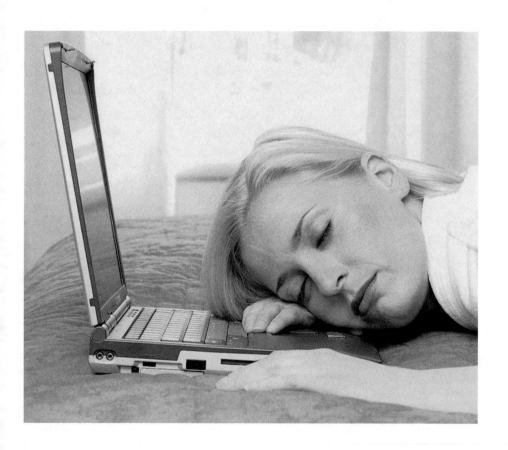

Hypnosis can be used to affect anything emotive and its resulting behaviours, beliefs and mental patterning.

Name a human emotional and it's resulting physical condition and chances are that someone somewhere has used hypnosis to create, alleviate, increase, reduce or change it.

Stress, the effects of trauma, both physical and emotional pain such as in childbirth, motivation, memory, breast and penis enlargement, and weight regulation, sexual, relationship, educational repair and enhancement, and even time travel in the form of past life regression and future life progression are just a few things that spring to mind.

Physiologically, even if hypnosis can't totally eradicate something it can and does go a long way in changing attitude and perception so that the body's healing process can act with less interruption.

I do think it rather sad though that such an amazing and awesome process which can produce such astonishing experience has, thanks to the unfortunate and often very lucrative focus of so many therapists, been almost exclusively associated with stopping smoking and weight loss.

At the Academy of Hypnotic Arts we target personal development and enhancement and the metaphysical market, areas which are badly under-investigated and serviced usually only by complex and cumbersome methods most of which have or had hypnosis as a basis.

Hypnosis can remove limiting beliefs, and ensure natural and learned abilities can be used with accuracy and consistency, but whatever that thing is called talent, you'll need that to be 'brilliant'.

Personal performance in business, sports, and relationships can all benefit from hypnosis. Even the best of us can suffer from limiting and blocking beliefs and emotions. On the field of play, whether that's a soccer pitch, an office, or even a bed. It's a fact that the removal of those limits will increase the enjoyment of doing and the achievement of succeeding.

Hypnosis can also be used purely for its entertainment value. Increasing and expanding the experience of life's wonders or as a holiday and a break from mundane experience.

Bettering recall, controlling stress, increasing creativity, self belief and image.

Our drives are emotional, and the whole point of our existence is one of our experience of the world, and the resulting use and movement of energy under this heading. Therefore, as well as saying that hypnosis could be used for **anything,** we can say that it should be tried on **everything.**

We truly are what we think, and hypnosis is the ultimate way of thinking the way we want to and have the right to, so we become what we truly deserve to be.

However lets look at one or two fabulous claims and put some perspective on them. Breast and penis enlargement. Both of these have had some success. Largely due to the following:

Breasts enlarge at certain times in life anyway. Certainly pregnancy causes this, but then so does the menstrual cycle in many women. Muscle tone helps, so focusing on the breast area can often lead to a general perk up just because the pects develop. Enlarging breasts in this way then can be done, but it isn't an exact science, and although a surgeon can predict both size and shape, the hypnotist can not. However the hypnotist can predict the absence of scar tissue and rejection problems. And there will be no chance of death caused by anesthetic drugs.

Penis size is about blood flow. Better the blood flow, better the size both in girth and length. Blood flow is affected by physical, neutritional and by emotional states. IF we can affect all of these we can often affect the penis.

The thing is the vast majority of seventeen year old guys are very happy about the size of their well behaving appendage and are never going to come to you seeking abundance. No, the vast majority of guys seeking a bigger better booster are fat middle aged neurotics with the diet of an alcoholic rat and the blood flow of the streets of central Pacville at rush hour.

Now these guys we can help. Just relieving the anxiety their diminishing reserves are causing will useually add the odd inch or so. And that can happen instantly. I know one guy who used Chinosis to do just that with very satisfying results. The rest can be achieved by instilling the desire to eat and exercise.

Some of the other stuff which I have yet to see convincing evidence of success on though are genetic conditions. I don't think you can reverse or influence the genetic blueprint we all have.

The fact is that I have never seen anyone able to change the shape or size of an ear, nose or the lips. I've yet to meet a hypnotist or victim whose hair has grown back, except when the loss was due to illness or anxiety. And no one has thus yet managed to get anyone to grow taller to my knowledge.

Cancers have been positively affected by suggestion and I think that is because some tumors are the body following a self-destruct command from the mind, and the above release of the bodies own healing process from the constraints of emotional prison.

I live in hope that some bright spark will come along and prove me wrong that we can't 'cure' everything.

I'm still waiting.

Hypnotic Phenomena:
Recognition And Testing

How do you know if you or anyone else is hypnotised?

You Test

Even an old hand like me who has developed a hypnotist sense for when people are in trance can sometimes miss it. So we look for phenomena that we would expect to see and then test that what we are observing is *in fact* what we are observing, just in case.

In accepted understanding the word 'trance' describes a profound change in both psychological attention and physiological condition.

In plainer language your conscious drifts off somewhere or is bypassed and certain predictable and observable changes happen to your body. Often, although by no means always, including relaxation. If your model or pattern for hypnosis includes the idea that it is relaxation, or if the hypnotist is suggesting that you become relaxed and you are accepting those suggestions, being relaxed is then almost certain to occur.

The thing to remember is that this is an **induced** state brought on as a reaction to suggestion. So 'trance' is not hypnosis, just a symptom of it.

One thing is certain, hypnotically induced 'trance' has no real comparison in the average experience other than when we are experiencing times of overwhelming emotion.

So how do we know when someone is hypnotised? To describe what you feel when in the presence of someone hypnotised is impossible, and not entirely necessary. I have seen people recognise whether volunteers in a stage show have 'gone' or not hundreds of times. It's instinctive so you would probably be able to 'tell' if someone was 'under' or not.

In saying that, certain phenomena often occurs spontaneously, and it's useful to know what these can be.

REM: Rapid eye movement. There is a 'batting' up and down movement of the eyelids and quick movement of the eyeball as occurs in dream sleep.

Blush: A lot of people blush when hypnotised, especially around the neck and face. In some cases you'll find that there is a slight quickening of heart rate and the blush would then be explained by the increased blood flow. On the other hand hypnosis is a state where the emotive mind is dominant and blushing is often caused by being emotive. Just watch someone embarrassed or very angry and you'll see emotive blushing.

Physical disassociation: If you lift a hypnotised persons hand and arm they won't withdraw. If you let the hand go it will either just collapse or just as likely stay where it is put. As an experiment try giving them quite a vigorous pinch, this will not elicit a yelp, flinch or any reaction, even if you don't suggest that the hand is numb or 'dead'. However, make sure they are hypnotised when you do this or it could earn you a slap.

Other things you may witness as spontaneous may be a dropping of the head, deeper breathing and a general flaccidity of posture. If they think this is what hypnosis is then this is what you will get. Obviously if they are hypnotised and are accepting your directions then you will see all of these and more if you suggest them.

There is however one phenomenon which remains, as far as I can see, consistent throughout the people I have hypnotised, they don't do a lot, they virtually freeze. No, I don't mean they get very cold, often body temperature rises, but, apart from the usual breathing and maybe and odd muscle spasm - they stop moving.

Most of the twitches and movement they would normally display simply go away. It's only when you get their mind focused on something emotional that these natural twitches are replaced by significantly individualistic movements that they didn't display before. We call these ideo-muscular responses or IMRs. And there are some hypnotic techniques which specifically use these movements to find out what the mind is doing. Personally I prefer to tell the mind to control the language centre of the brain and just ask it questions.

If I do use IMR I keep it simple. Naturally occurring IMRs include nodding and shaking their head and smiling. So saying, "nod your head if you understand," is a lot more natural than asking for a finger to lift to say yes or no. If you like IMRs fine. But there is absolutely no reason to use them other than using muscle testing as a convincer. We'll talk about that later.

All of the above things or none of them may be observed during a session, but don't worry if you don't see them. Visual interpretation isn't always the best judge of whether you've obtained hypnosis or not. What you feel is just as important as what you see.

Throughout this book you'll be reminded that your instinct and intent are the most important tools as a hypnotist. If you are sure they are hypnotised then, chances are, they are. And when they are sure, they will be hypnotised.

In a moment I will tell you how to test during the session but as with anything hindsight is wonderful and it's always easier to check things after the event. Post hypnotic phenomena nearly always include:

Time distortion: It's quite common for hypnotised people to have no idea of the length of time they have been hypnotised. Sometimes even after a twenty minute session there's a conviction that nothing has occurred at all and you get asked to get on with it. I've had people who refused to pay because they didn't think anything had happened. So, I had to re-hypnotise them and make sure they **knew.**

Partial or full memory loss: In consultation this occurs in nearly all people, the odd exception is usually because of the way the state has been managed or ended. They may remember the general context of the session or the odd bit of what you do. Or they may remember nothing at all. I usually tell them to bring back anything they feel is important but this hasn't in my experience increased the numbers who do recall content.

We are not talking about suggested events here but totally spontaneous ones. These things happen all on their own without any help from you.

There is one phenomenon that if not present you have not got a workable state of hypnosis even if you have all of the above in spades.

Acceptance of suggestion:

Hypnosis has to include the unquestioning acceptance of suggestion and direction. If this is not in place you may have all sorts of states but not hypnosis and you would be less than useless on a hypnotic level anyway. If they don't accept your suggestions, directions, or guidance then they may as well be talking to the bloke down the pub.

The early fathers of hypnosis at the turn of the 20th century regularly tested hypnosis by using physical catalepsy or the inability to consciously move a limb. This is easily tested by 'sticking' a hand to the furniture, telling the hypnotee that they were unable to stand up – effectively sticking them to a chair, or by performing some kind of deliberate catalepsy such as being unable to lift or bend an arm.

Milton Erickson was fond of using visual hallucinations as a way of testing suggestion and of convincing hypnotees that they were hypnotised. A favourite of his was telling them that there was a dog sitting next to them, or that someone in the room had disappeared.

These are excellent tests. Please don't be put off using them by their seeming to be playing with someone's mind. If you don't test and do analysis then you are just playing and the result of failure will be far worse.

Hypnotherapy in general now disregards these things claiming they are 'tricks' only to be done on stage by disreputable hypnotists who don't really understand the subject. The truth is that if you can't do these things then you can't actually hypnotise, and you most certainly wouldn't be able to use these 'tricks' if you didn't understand the subject.

Without acceptance of these suggestions you are doing nothing more than relaxo clinical psychology or psychotherapy which has an abysmal success rate at best.

So test

A few good tests have been mentioned above but here's a couple more.

From Barry Thain – clinical hypnotist – tell your client that when you clap your hands the room will become dark. Tell them to open their eyes and clap. If the suggestion works watch their pupils which should enlarge as if in a real dark room.

Tell the hypnotee that when they open their eyes and talk to you their arm will rise and float and they won't notice.

Basically you test hypnosis and the acceptance of suggestion and seeing if those suggestions are accepted and followed. What that suggestion is should in my mind be instantly observable. So for preference, make it physical.

Real Rapport

In many hypnosis and influence books, certainly those written post NLP, a lot of time and effort is spent on explaining how to build and obtain rapport, which according to dictionary.com is:

RAPPORT:
Relationship, especially one of mutual trust or emotional affinity.

So rapport is basically being friends.

Over the last three decades a lot of observation and research has been done on this subject. As a result it has been deduced that people in a state of rapport mirror each other taking up similar stances and positions. They speak using similar terminology such as visual or auditory or kinesthetic as in feelings, and they match each other in most – if not all ways

The theory of 'establishing rapport' then goes that if you deliberately copy or mirror your target, as well as using words they will resonate with, such as "see" for a visual, "Hear" for an auditory and "Feel" for a kinesthetic person, that this will create rapport.

What is being observed here, though, is the result or the symptoms of rapport, not the reasons for it. Thinking that people who share symptoms should have the same condition is like expecting two people who cough to have bronchitis, although one has lung cancer and the other tuberculosis. Similar symptoms do not produce the same disease. Two women wearing the same evening gown does not always build rapport, well not of the nice friendly kind anyway.

The thing is that after watching lots of seminars, reading tons of books, experimenting with all sorts of ideas, and most importantly observing the so-called experts, one has come to a single opinion… The only people for whom this works are those who believe it will, those who have been hypnotically patterned to react in certain ways when those patterns are fired. If they have **any** doubt that these rapport building methods work, they don't. They do however piss people off when they are confronted by someone mimicking them.

In real rapport a form of communication is being unleashed which will inevitably become an event which may or may not result in the above physical conditions. But it will result in what we can use as a connection between two people. It verges on the telepathic and is always entirely empathetic, and always non-conscious and automatic. You just know how the other person feels; you don't have to think about it.

How that is achieved is neither a science nor even an art. It isn't something you can practice and learn, it's below and beyond that. It is however something that you can turn on. Just like charm. The easiest way of achieving this is so amazingly simple it has been sadly overlooked for several decades, and that involves people liking people.

Real Rapport happens when people like each other. The accepted theory among established rapport experts is that "People like people like them".

This frankly is incredibly short sighted and quite simply wrong. Take a look at any professional soccer game in England, especially 'Local Derby' games. Here you have two teams from the same city. All the opposing fans speak much the same dialect, work often in the same places, and attend the same social venues and schools. They shop in the same shops, dress the same, and so on.

They are mirroring each other almost exactly in both physical and emotional states and moods and according to the theory that people like people who are like them, they should be in rapport. Yet most Saturdays, were it not for the police presence, they would quite happily tear each other limb from limb. Sadly, sometimes they do so despite the police.

Now look at the fat, dumpy, height and thinking challenged Hobbit at the hypnosis show who is meeting the Adonis like, tall, handsome hypnotist superstar and, despite the outward and indeed inward differences, real rapport occurs. The fan likes the God like performer. And the hypnotist likes the fans adoration and therefore the fan. That's real rapport.

Of course I do know the above is true as I've been there many times.

Now run through the number of couples you know who are "like chalk and cheese". Those people who are together in the ultimate rapport not *because* of their similarities but despite them. I know quite a few and so has anyone else I've asked to try this.

For this reason I don't accept the premise that people just like people who are **like** them and have my own phrase for understanding Real Rapport.

"People like people who **like them**."

It's instinctive. We are attracted to people who like us and to people who give off all the signals of being comfortable and happy with us. It goes way beyond the external, way beyond consciousness. It even goes beyond reasoning and quite possibly beyond, or at least behind our current understanding of what communication is. It's something that just happens. And we can trust that much more than something we are deliberately trying for. Although we can turn it on deliberately, the best thing to do then is forget it.

How do we do this? If you want someone to like and trust you, all you have to do is like and trust them. This has to be natural and easy. The second that conscious effort comes into play we will begin to doubt ourselves and people will sense it and give that doubt straight back to us.

Think of all the people you've met and connected with favourably in your life. I'll bet there was no conscious effort needed to make those real friends who not only seem happy with who they are but just as importantly are happy with who you are.

Now think of those you just couldn't get along with no matter what. Are there any redeeming factors you can think of? Of course there are but you still don't like them. You don't like them and that's where it ends – no rapport. And that's okay if the target is just making friends, you can't be friends with everyone, it's too expensive at Christmas.

However if it's really important that you want to and need to have rapport with someone then all you need to do is find something you like about them and concentrate on that. If it's their hair then think about how nice that is. If it's their demeanour, their speech pattern, their nose, their choice of tie or even just the fact that they are speaking with you. Find something you like and allow them to become, at least for a while in your reality, that thing. If you like them, or an aspect of them, then they will, with no effort at all, like you or an aspect of you. And that my friend is rapport.

As a working hypnotist though it is important to have a connection sometimes with people you wouldn't be friends with. It just isn't necessary to **build** one. If they accept you as a hypnotist, and you accept you in that role, the rapport just happens. I've seen it a million times. It's rapport built of respect or even fear, but it is still rapport. That is a relationship where the end result is a common goal – and how can you not like someone who shares your goals? It's what I think of as EXPERT rapport.

We all experience this with our doctors, legal advisors, business peers and those we aspire to become. As children we get it with almost every adult, and certainly as a hypnotist you will find it no problem to feel and use this very special asset of just being what you are.

You don't need to learn how to do this. If you're confident in your capabilities of hypnotising it happens. It's like breathing; and just like breathing if you try and become conscious with it, it suddenly becomes hard to do. I suggest that you trust it to work just as you trust your body to suck and blow air. Providing you have every faith and confidence in your ability and skill to provide what they are paying you for and so exude confidence, rapport happens the moment you announce your credentials. And is cemented in the reality of your intent – you just have to believe it's going to work.

Now if that isn't enough for you to trust your own natural rapport building talents, then you are in the money. You also have another rapport producing thing going for you as a Hypnotist rather than a road sweeper, and that is what I call the **Awe Rapport.**

The moment you announce you are a hypnotist a lot of people will immediately hold you in awe. That's not just a mixture of respect and fear, but something much deeper that goes back before we knew what history was. It is the same tribal connection that the

B A Hypnotist

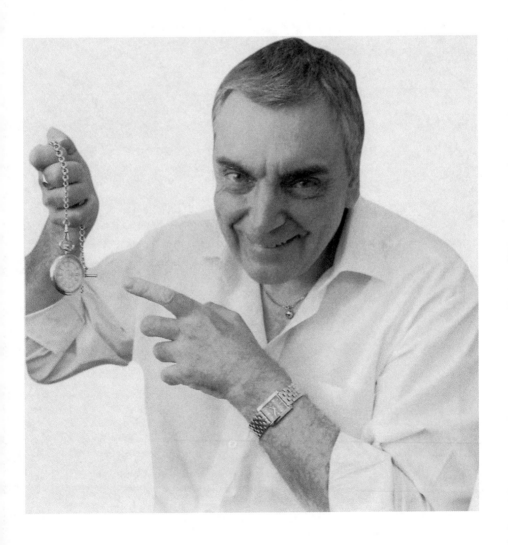

For this part of the book I'm going to assume you are reading this from the point of someone who intends working with hypnosis not just playing with it, either as a career – retirement supplement – part time income – vocation - as a supplement to your current occupation... whatever.

That doesn't mean you can't use it if it's not your job, just that I need to know where to point the book. So I'm imagining that you need to know what to do in a hypnosis consultation whether that be in an office or elsewhere as opposed to just banging someone under the influence down the pub and sticking them to something or someone. That particular skill is already covered anyway in my other book entitled "Deeper and Deeper – the secrets of stage hypnosis.

For the purposes of **this** book we will assume that you are a hypnotist, not a trick cyclist. We'll also assume that you and I are in agreement as to what that word means. If not, I will quite happily see you at a conference, on a radio or TV show, or an Internet discussion group, anytime, anywhere.

So let's start at the very beginning. I'm not going to lay down rules, that's not how I work. And if you are really in tune with yourself it shouldn't be how you work either. This is how I do things. Some of it will work for you. Some other bits of it will still work for you but you won't try them because it doesn't feel right, and the rest should never be done by someone other than me because I don't want the competition.

The thing is that hypnosis, above anything else, is an art. And I will show you how to use that way just as the originators of the talent did.

I'll show you how to mix the paint, how to hold the brush and maybe even suggest what you paint, but the rest is up to you. You are after all your own artist. I can say one thing however. All of this stuff works.

Hypnosis **actually** begins when you know you are a hypnotist. Hypnosis **apparently** begins when you tell someone you're a hypnotist. It's then you'll more than likely hear the immortal phrase we took to title this work with,
"He's a hypnotist. Don't look in his eyes!"

This is often followed by the most stupid question ever,
"Can you make me cluck like a chicken?"
My stock answer is of course
"Yes, but why would you want me to?"

Initial Meeting
And Pre-talk

In the beginning there was the word, and the word was **Hypnosis**.

I tell people I am a **hypnotist** and so people come to me expecting, and rightfully so, to be **hypnotised**.

I don't call myself a hypno-anything such as a therapist or analyst because they have a lot to do with psychotherapy, psychology and often very little to do with hypnosis. Over the years a lot of my clients have made the point that it's because of my being a straight forward hypnotist that they have come to me. They don't want to be therapised, they do want to be hypnotised.

Now as I've said I can sometimes fail, so I'll initially make an appointment to see how good a hypnotic subject they are and how responsive they are to **my** methods. I'll also tell them that with those who are responsive that my success rate is 100% because this is true. I have successfully hypnotised 100% of those who I have successfully hypnotised. Which is a lot and enough.

Most schools of therapy would now tell you that it is vital in the initial appointment to tell the client all you know about hypnosis and to establish what they know, what they expect and so forth. It's also apparently vitally important to make tons of notes and get a complete medical, family, educational, genetic breakdown and if possible discover what they had for breakfast on the sixth of June 2004.

Personally I just talk to them for while. I will make an effort to discover what they are passionate about and what they expect to be able to do or not do at the end of the session.

I'll agree that understanding what they know hypnosis is and what they are expecting is indeed very important. The first thing I always do is establish what the person I'm working with thinks hypnosis is. Whatever this is that's what I say I'll give them. I then ignore that and hypnotise them. The only reason I need to know what they think they may experience is to be able to recognise it when they do.

Most people over the age of four have an idea of what hypnosis is. I had to smile when my god son Michael stood in front of me at that age swinging a plastic toy clock on a length of string saying "Your eyes are getting sleepy…".

If they think it's relaxation then often they'll experience relaxation. If they think it's sleep then they'll get an approximation – if they expect that and then snore I've been too successful. If they don't have a definite preset idea then great I'll just go where I feel is right, which is what I do anyway, and usually what happens to them. Providing those patterns don't interfere with your aim then why bother changing them? I'm not into educating clients as the vast majority don't want that. They want their patterning sorted and that done using hypnosis.

I don't do therapy, NLP or Umbagumba. I do Coach Chinosis which is only another way of presenting hypnosis and symbolism, and wearing my other hat I do Mentoring and Coaching but always the basis is of what I do is hypnosis and not psychotherapy and I am always clear about that.

So, we'll take it that they have in some way contacted me and that we are together for the first meeting. I don't bother to ask too many questions at this point, as a Hypnotist I don't need to. If anything I'll just chat, about the weather if they are British and about the weather if they are not. It's a point of reference we all share as the damn stuff is everywhere. Listen to how the weather is making them feel as that gives you an idea of how they are based today. Listen for terms such as miserable rain or overbearing heat, sure signs of the miseries.

Then I find I don't do much at all but listen for a while. If they are there for some remedial work they will tell you most things – even the ones you didn't need to know. If they are there for personal performance they will tell you most things – even the ones you didn't need to know. I guess people equate hypnotists with priests and doctors because as soon as they know what you do it opens the floodgates to their very private worlds.

I regularly get whole life stories at the drop of the word hypnosis, on trains, planes, in swimming pools and cafés. Thankfully they also do so in the consultation room which gives us a chance to understand their passions, and understanding their passions is much more important than having their medical record.

So, I am listening to what they say and joining them in their reality. That's where we are going to work. I never question why they have come or attempt to diagnose their condition. To do that I'd need the proper training and machinery for a physical condition, and for an emotional condition I know what the trouble is and am happy to leave them with their preferred label.

Their 'problem' is always inappropriate or unproductive patterns of belief and behaviour. That is all I've seen in three decades apart from physical trauma, and the inappropriate or unproductive patterns of belief and behaviour that accompanies that. And when you take away the labels for the symptoms that is all you will ever see.

I'll let this chat go on until one of two things occur… they stop talking or I get bored. I usually get bored before they stop talking so I just interrupt and say

"Okay, let's **do** something."

I am doing a couple of really important things here. Number one I'm getting on with it and number two I am telling them that we will **do** something.

From the moment they accept you as a hypnotist, every word becomes a suggestion. **Don't give their mind a choice**, it may not go the way you would like.

NOTE: "Let's DO something". I don't say lets try something as that implies that there could be an unpredictable outcome. However if I say DO and nothing happens I have lost nothing as I will just act as if the nothing was exactly what should have happened in the first place. I know what that should be but they don't, so it can go differently to expectations without their knowing it.

Think of this rather like a magician. If they just tell you to watch their hand and at the first pass they fail to get the card from the secret pocket all they will do is show you the empty hand and then make the pass again and voila, there's the card. As far as you the observer is concerned they didn't cock it up the first time because you had no idea what the target was.

At this point there is no mention of 'hypnotising' either, even though I know that's what is happening and guess they do too at some place in their mind. After all it is what they are here for.

There's a good reason for not telling them I'm going to hypnotise them and that is that I may not be going to use the best induction for them. Or for me.

If I don't use one that appeals to their mind, or if I'm not firing on all cylinders, there is an outside possibility that the chosen induction doesn't work. On the odd occasion that happens I haven't failed in their eyes because there is no "Right this is where we hypnotise you", and no suggestion of failure has therefore taken place.

If it doesn't work I'll just smile and say,
"That's interesting." And move right on to another induction still not telling them that this is what's happening. Unless they have had previous experience then they won't know what's happening. This is useful with analytical people because you don't give them actually anything to analyse. And it's very beneficial for those who are scared as you are not giving them anything to be scared of.

Sometimes I'll take this approach and speed it up to the point where my whole pre-talk boils down to this...

"What do you know about hypnosis? You're wrong. Just close your eyes. . ." and induce. This works well as a confusion or shock induction and if it fails I just go "That's interesting" and go back to the full asking what they think hypnosis really is.

Don't worry if you've been taught a more clinical approach and feel you need to take their name and address, inside leg measurement, full medical record and everything else about them - you can do that later, you don't need those details in the UK anyway other than for insurance purposes and marketing and this feeling of needing the bits of paper will pass as you become a more direct and rapid worker.

Rapid, Intense Hypnotic Inductions

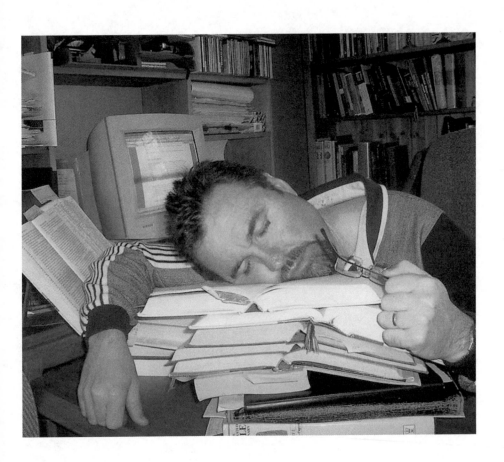

Hypnotic induction rituals don't have to take a long time. Read the chapter heading.

One of the basic differences between hypnosis and hypnotherapy is that the aim of the hypnotist is to do this quickly and intensely.

I could have said instantly because hypnosis always happens instantly – you either are or you are not and there is therefore always a point of hypnosis. People in the hypnotic establishment get quite upset with me when I question why you need to take twenty minutes to relax someone when you could hypnotise them in much less than a minute, and I'm not writing this book to upset people. So I won't ask that question. Much.

Over the years there have been a tremendous number of differing techniques developed and invented to induce hypnosis. Some immensely complex or just time consuming, some elegant and beautiful and then the lot I favour – simple and productive.

I work on the fact that you can have too much of a good thing and have often seen people fail before they have begun. Not just because of the induction they used, but because they couldn't make their mind up which one to use out of the thousands of possibilities out there.

A quick Google search using the term "Hypnosis induction script" just landed 105,000 pages.

The fact is you don't need loads. I work almost entirely with three, all of which I can do in my sleep, or their sleep (hypnosis gag), with no thought other than doing it.

For that reason in this book I'm going to give you just a few, and hope you can get really good at one or two, to the point where they come so naturally and simply to you that you won't need any others. Hopefully you will develop your own variation as that is when you will become really good, at least at the induction.

I won't pay too much attention to eye fixation or swinging watches, which I use on occasion, or to bi-neural beat software. All of which sing the same tune, "When this happens – this results". It's what we hypnotists tend to call a **suggestion** and quite honestly hypnosis doesn't work any better with them. It's like a magician. Anyone can go out and buy and perform a 'trick', but the best magicians can use anything to hand to perform. They don't need the box or silk, just the knowledge.

I have found that the simpler you make it, the easier it is for both parties, even groups, to get the state rapidly and as intensely as those seen on stage.

It's misleading to think in terms of depth and levels of hypnosis, intensity and fine tuning is much more accurate. No one is going into or down anywhere, although I do use these words for those who tell me that is what they are expecting. And sometimes just through sheer force of habit which a wonderful thing to cultivate.

The habit of hypnotising.

Some of the inductions I'm about to give you appear in my stage hypnosis book. This isn't because of laziness, but because the fact is that they do not change wherever I do them, and shouldn't change for you either. I've found these work for most people and have yet to be convinced that one is particularly better than another.

Some of them were invented somewhere by the unknown hypnotist and some were perfected by people like Erickson or much earlier by Braid and work just fine. I am not aware of where they all originate, and when you read the books, neither is anyone else. It doesn't matter.

I drive a car but have no idea who designed it or the name of the guy who discovered how to refine the petrol I put in it, but it still gets me out and about okay.

I have mostly refined and changed these inductions myself anyway, as have others before me, so you are getting hybrids which you will undoubtedly add to or subtract from yourself. I claim no real invention here, but lots and lots of usage.

Don't get stuck in the belief that different types of folk need different inductions or that different circumstances need differing approaches. The induction should fit **you** as much as it does them, if not more so. And the smoother and more confident you can be the better.

If you are worrying about which of the hundred and five thousand inductions you should use you will never perfect *your* approach or technique so I suggest you don't go overboard in gathering them.

The most important thing is that you believe in the ones you use and that you do not have to read them.

These are not all stage inductions; they don't have the dramatic impact needed to entertain. Not one of them needs any 'special' conditions. No comfortable chair, therapist's couch, subdued lighting or even a room.

If you can't do your chosen inductions at the drop of a hat in any situation, time or place with the success rate of around 80%, then you need more practice. Or more probably, it will pay you to train in hypnosis so that your technique can be fine-tuned by someone with experience. Although this book can tell you it can't show you.

The fathers of hypnosis didn't have need for gadgets – excepting of course candles, swinging watches or jewelled pendants and other handy tools to get and sustain the recipients' attention, and if we believe only half their written records they still had a success rate beyond belief in comparison to today's, and dealt with mental and physical conditions most hypnotherapists wouldn't go anywhere near, and which many schools will say are contra-indicated - whatever that means.

To be fair, this is as much because of fear of the legal system and of upsetting the established medical profession than it is anything else. It's because of this and the watered down and over-analysed and intellectualised approaches in use and being taught at the moment that hypnosis has lost its cutting edge and metaphysical magic.

What contra-indicated actually means is that the person using the phrase has been told by people who failed, that hypnosis won't work in such and such a case. I find this happens when the person making this assumption hasn't got the skills to make it work and therefore presumes no one else can.

It's the "If I can't do it then neither can you" syndrome.

All you need to get the following inductions to work for you is the belief and assurance that they will and someone to do them with.

Inductions

The main inductive process has already taken place and that is, quite simply, their knowing that you can induce. I've seen it dozens of times where just introducing myself as a hypnotist has caused that glazed over look in their eyes. And, with a little practice and experience you will be able to use that point to suggest real hypnosis apparently instantly.

No, that isn't a special trick as all hypnosis is instant. There is a point when you ain't followed very quickly by a point where you is.

For now however we'll look at the expected rituals which we call hypnotic induction, after all this what the bulk of your victims will expect.

While clicking your fingers and saying sleep will work with around 20% of the people you meet it helps to focus you and your hypnotee, and excites the model of hypnosis in both your minds if you use some sort of ritualistic process to get hypnosis.

As far as inductions are concerned the truth is that there is no such thing as 'Stage' hypnosis or hypno 'therapy'. These describe where the art is being done and the target it is being used for but not what it is.

Hypnosis is hypnosis, and an induction is anything that produces that state.

Hypnosis, regardless of the approach or technique you decide to use, requires that your hypnotees are using their creative abilities and have, for the moment, put aside any limiting factor supplied by their conscious brain, allowing them to accept your suggestions by focusing their mind on you and you alone. They have a single thought and that is focused internally and is guided by you. That doesn't mean that the mind or subconscious doesn't make choices. Of course it can. And as you'll see when we discuss suggestion, it's up to you what those choices are. It just means that for the time they are hypnotised only the internal reality is important.

Hypnosis, we must remember, is a state of mind. And contrary to what the established accepted theories say, it is a state of mind solely controlled and directed by the hypnotist. The state itself is therefore mostly what you make it.

Although your hypnotee may expect to experience a state reminiscent of sleep, it is not necessary. In saying that, relaxation has become a recognisable part of hypnosis because it is the expected symptom of the state in the minds of most people – even most hypnotists, not everyone however experiences the relaxed 'trance' which is always suggested by the hypnotist. Hypnosis does not **need** it.

You do not need it; however, unless they tell you otherwise, that is usually what your hypnotee has paid for. And if that is what they want, then that is, to a point, what they are going to get. You as 'The Hypnotist' must know that relaxation isn't the cause of the hypnotic state; it's just a symptom of suggestion. Once they have accepted a suggestion to the degree where they are experiencing what they expected then they will accept ninety nine percent of all your suggestions if you formulate them correctly.

Induce means to cajole, persuade, to lead. You've already done that if you ask them to close their eyes and they do. The rest is setting up the path of communication and fine tuning this to its best wavelength.

Even so, for the purposes of this book, I'm going to give you some approaches which are easy to remember, rapid in effect and some have worked with millions of people for nearly two hundred years.

Learn these first by rote if you have to, and then by practice. It's *vital* that you know these, or your preferred version of them, inside out, and that you are comfortable and relaxed with what you do. Stumbling and stopping while you try to remember how this induction goes, or that one, will do nothing to help, so when using these just go with the way they flow from you. There are no prizes for being word perfect.

[Note: you can hypnotise the more suggestible by reading these but if you start that way you'll find it much harder to make the transition to not reading. So don't do it.]

Whatever you do don't fall for the old myth that you need a different induction for every personality type out there. It's a lie. On the whole I use the eye lock or magnetic hands in one on one. I use the arm lift or magnetic hands or eye fixation when demonstrating or exhibiting, usually a combination of all of these. And on stage I use the very dramatic drop back or chair drop.

Basically that's five inductions. These work with almost everyone I hypnotise because I am good at them, damn good. I know them inside out. They never alter except for minor variations of mood from me. No matter who I am using them on I never falter and have complete confidence because I'm not wondering whether I've picked the right induction for this or that person.

Just as Rohypnol works predictably so do these inductions. You can of course vary them to fit you, but just get good at what works for you. Get damn good.

If you've read my stage book you will see lots of similarities here, with some minor tweaks to fit the point of this book. That's because I really do use these same inductions and very little else. The reason for this is of course that when you become really adept at something you don't need a million other ways to achieve the same ends. The idea that everyone or every type of person needs a different approach is rubbish.

Eye Lock

This is my version of the old eye closure induction made famous by the American hypnotist Dave Elman but mentioned in books a hundred years before: this is by far one of the easiest inductions and the one I tend to use first in virtually all circumstances apart from on stage.

It's up to you whether you do this with them seated or standing.

You:
"Close your eyes and pretend, just imagine that your eyes won't open. And when you're positive, when you are absolutely certain that your eyes won't open, test them."

What should happen now is that you will see them lifting their eyebrows and really struggling to get their eyes open, this can take a while sometimes as long as ten seconds, never rush them or interrupt the emergence of the mind.

Sometimes of course, they will misinterpret what you say and just open them. When this happens, say:
"No. I said to test that your eyes won't open – you're testing that they will. We know that they will. But we need to imagine that they won't. Let's do this again."

Repeat the first part and more often than not, I have a 99% success rate with this, they won't be able to open them. Now remember the big secret of hypnosis: if they will accept one suggestion they'll accept them all. Say to them,
"Great. Now allow that feeling to travel from your eyelids up through your forehead, down through your neck and shoulders,

through your arms to your fingertips, through your torso, your abdomen, down through your legs and feet and into the floor. And just let go"

It is my belief that when the target of the hypnotee being unable to open their eyes by will is achieved, you have mind or subconscious dominance, as it is only in the capabilities of the creative mind to believe an illogical scenario such as their eyes being 'stuck' shut. If you have that then you have hypnosis.

This is a combination of a progressive relaxation and the eye closure. I don't always do it this way but when I do it definitely increases the intensity of the communication.

I've also made downward passes with my hands when it feels right, a very old thing and one that works. And I always look at the bit of their body I'm referring to. I'm sure this helps because they **will** know. The mind is brilliant at picking these things up from the sensory equipment which the brain usually ignores.

At this point they will relax. I've rarely seen them not do this. As I've said, the relaxation thing is deeply embedded in the zeitgeist, that is, in the universal conscious we all share.

Magnetic hands

Although I use this in any situation it is my favourite with groups as it gives you a wonderful physical indication of where people are and allows you to pace yourself with more than the individual.

Although at first impression it may look like another physically based test, this induction does not rely on predictable muscle movement and only works if the psychic compliance is there and imagination is working. At once it is not only an elegant induction it is also a great convincer for the mind.

Have them sit. Get them to put their hands out in front of themselves with their elbows bent and their fingers together outstretched, palms facing each other with a gap of about 6 inches between them. Make sure they don't rest their arms or elbows on their lap or the arms of chair as they need free movement.

Tell them to close their eyes, this helps their concentration and stops visual distraction and once again it is expected.

Now begin to suggest that their hands are being pulled together by magnets, getting closer and closer. I actually reach forward and 'place' magnets in their hands.

"Now your hands are being irresistibly drawn together and, at the moment, the very instant they touch you will feel a huge wave of comfort, peace and calm spread through every nerve, muscle and fibre. The moment your fingers touch your hands will fall gently into your lap and your heavy head will drop forward as you enter a wonderfully calm and peaceful state."

This can take a long time – up to 2 minutes with some people; however if you have too you can quicken the process a little.

Watch them carefully and, providing you have some movement of the hands toward each other, wait until the hands are an inch or two apart and then quickly slap them together pulling slightly forward and down. Push them firmly into their laps at the same time in a commanding voice, say,
"Go."

This is what we refer to as a shock induction. Shock inductions work this way...

The target is to turn the logic off and to create a state of emotional and creative (mind) dominance. This always happens when confusion or fear happens. Simply put the brain can't handle these. They don't make sense; there is no logic to fear and confusion. So, the brain being a slow inadequate organ of reasoning and process it gives up and gives over control to the much faster and less cumbersome mind. Mind just reacts. It does choose but it doesn't reason or apply logic to those choices.

So with the mind being an excepting and reactive beast it will accept the suggestion to "Go!" when it gets it. You could also of course command "Sleep", "Relax", or "Zap!" – they'll all work because the creative and emotive mind is already expecting to be hypnotised.

Wrist Lift

At an exhibition we were doing in London some years ago a clinical hypnotist Barry Thain was talking about a wrist lift induction he used. I totally misunderstood him but that night came up with what I thought was his wrist induction… turns out it was mine.

Again this includes both induction and test for suggestion acceptance. By far the easiest way to work.

Sit at the side of the client and take the wrist and arm closest to you. Don't worry about touching people, if they shook your hand when they came in they won't bother with you holding their wrist. If you do the standard thing and ask if they mind being touched then they could just begin to wonder what it was you were going to touch. If the touch is harmless don't give it the potential for harm – remember every word is a suggestion.

Now tell them to give you their arm. Don't command but do be firm. Hold their wrist in one hand and their elbow in another and say,
"Give me your arm."

If you don't feel the full weight of their lower arm and can't move the elbow freely they haven't given you the arm, they are allowing you to hold it. Insist that they give you the arm until you are holding the arm up by the wrist, their hand becomes flaccid and that when you move the elbow there is no resistance. At this point move the arm into a subtly different position from the one they gave it to you. This tells their mind that you are in control of what happens to the arm not them.

At this point tell them to close their eyes. I mostly close their eyes because it's expected and because it's an easy way of cutting out distraction. I do induce with eye fixation but prefer the eye closed thing, remember the induction should fit you as well. I have done this induction with their eyes open but only to show off in class. I don't see the point otherwise.

Now say,

"That's right. Now your arm is floating. It's not going up and it isn't going down. It's just staying there, floating just where it is, not moving. That's right."

You may have to repeat this a few times.

While you are speaking pay attention to how heavy the arm is and to the hand. What you are looking for is two things. First the hand remains perfectly flaccid with no tension or movement. Secondly the weight of the arm will go. Without moving up you'll feel that you are no longer holding the arm up and remarkably there will be no upward movement and usually little or no muscle rigidity around the elbow.

Slowly take your hand away and they will stay there quite happily for ages. I once did a full twenty-minute session with someone in my car in a McDonald's car park and his hand didn't move at all until I woke him. Apart from a little stiffness he reported nothing amiss with the arm. Interesting.

This induction allows me to do a great convincing test as well. When the arm just floats tell them it's your arm. It belongs to you and that no matter where you put it the arm will just stay there.

Now tell them to open their eyes while you position the arm in strange positions and ask them whose arm it is. If the arm is

94

doing what you wish they will say that it is your arm and then look slightly confused.

Don't worry, that's just the brain trying to figure out why it lost control of a limb.

When I'm satisfied I usually push the arm down into their lap and close their eyes and begin the next stage. The deepening.

Eye and Body Fixation

Fixation, or rather fascination has two effects. One, it focuses their mind on some action which is illogical and, as such, requires the mind to be dominant. It goes without saying that the logical brain can't handle illogical emotive stuff. And two, it shows you the acceptance of suggestion in the most easily of observable ways.

My favourite is the old staring at a bright light as we use on stage. This tires the eyes and helps the acceptance of the suggestion that they will close. And it also shows you how focused they are. Keep them there for a couple of minutes and although the tears are streaming and they obviously are desperate to close the eyes, they are stuck because you have told them to stare and not take their eyes away from the light.

At the same time you can use arm catalepsy. Simply raise the wrists up to their chest height and tell them to stay there. I've done a twenty minute session including 'waking' them up and chatting to them and the arms have stayed in that position.

It is also possible to induce by holding any object at a point in their line of sight just high enough for them to still see it without tilting their head back. Given a moment or two you will see their eyes begin to close and in another couple of minutes bang - away they go.

This sounds really impressive as you don't need to speak but it really isn't. You have already told them what and who you are. They have agreed to look at the thing without tilting their head back. In fact there are probably three or four other suggestion which have been accepted before the actual induction has been done.

'Deepening' the state

You can now 'deepen' the state they are in. As I've already said this is a myth.

There are no levels of hypnosis, there is just hypnosis. What you are actually doing when you 'deepen' is fine tuning and reinforcing the channel of communication. Enhancing the flow of energies between you and the hypnotee. It's a great opportunity for both of you to increase and intensify your focus. On the odd occasion I have used this deepening as an elongated induction and it worked perfectly well, even to the point of inducing others who could hear me.

Again I don't vary this, it works. There may be a million variations on this theme but trust me, it isn't what you do or say that is important to the hypnotee. It's how good you are at doing them.

This is how I do it, you can work your own method and I know this works because it has a few hundred thousand times.

When I first started in the game and wasn't so confident in my abilities I would sometimes drag this out to the point that some people ended up snoring. You can have confidence that this can be done quite quickly with the desired effect.

This deepener uses the physical things that will be happening and does not impose any visualisations or other stuff which is often the reason for people returning to their previous state. This is designed entirely to focus the mind internally on the mental and physical condition of the hypnotee and the voice and presence of the hypnotist.

"I'm going to begin counting, and with every number I go past, with every deep breath you take, with every firm beat of your heart, you are doubling the - - - - you are feeling now."

(This could be relaxation if they are obviously relaxed, it could be peace and calm which are my favorites or anything you 'feel' from the hypnotee.)

"There is only the sound of my voice and nothing else bothers or disturbs you. The only important sound is the sound of my voice and any other sound just serves to increase the feeling of peace and calm that you find invading every pore and fibre of your body and mind.

Ten. Deeper and deeper, nine, with every deep breath, eight, with every firm beat, seven with every number going deeper and deeper. More and more relaxed. Five,"

(Miss the number six to cause confusion and to strengthen the acceptance of a different state of focus. 'I missed a number and so must be becoming hypnotised') and so on down to one.

Note: I always count down to put them in; up to bring them out. There is no particular reason for this other than being consistent.

On the count of one I just get them to imagine a wonderful place and immediately start using their creative capabilities. There is neither reason nor point in compounding and repeating this. If you haven't got them now, you won't get them. At least not today.

Hypnosis 'Levels'

This was posted recently to our internet discussion forum by Jenny from Curvessynergy.com

"There are 2 levels of hypnosis. Hypnotised and Not-Hypnotised. There are zillions of *trance levels* though. Some of them include hypnosis." Jenny

I agree with this.

Hypnosis is a mental state not a building with floors and elevators; although these can be used as a metaphor for deepening or intensifying the state it's important that the hypnotist recognizes that these are mental energy patterns and not physical levels.

Spend too much time or expend too much energy and focus on achieving the correct 'level' of boredom or relaxation and you may easily lose control of the situation and then lose your connection.

Think of it like an electrical appliance with a cut off mechanism or a screensaver on your computer; spend too much time doing nothing and not moving energy and it just shuts down. So don't worry about levels, keep your connection.

The only working level is the one where they accept without question you're suggestions.

Intention

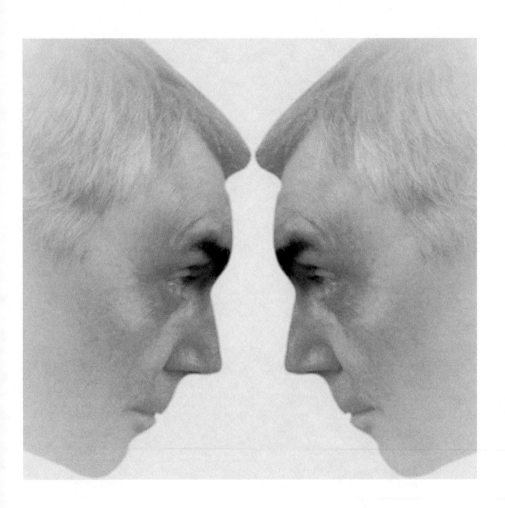

Without doubt the most important thing that a hypnotist must get right is the intention behind their work. Whatever you intend the result to be is almost certainly the result you will get.

This is true in every aspect of life. It isn't what you think do or say that gets the result; ultimately it's the intent behind all of that external stuff that really matters.

To demonstrate how important intent is I actually did some digging on my bookshelf and found some research done on one of the bedrocks of hypnotherapy which to me is amazingly scary in its short-sightedness. "People under hypnosis will not attempt to harm themselves or others."

In the book, "Modern Hypnosis", edited and compiled by Lesley Khun and Salvatore Russo Ph.D., 1970 edition published by the Wilshire Book Company, Library of Congress number 58:13449, there are two research summations, one from a guy called Lloyd W Roland Ph.D. and the other by the demi-god of hypnotherapy, Dr. Milton H Erickson.

Now the first experiment was entitled "Will hypnotised persons try to harm themselves or others?" and the second is named "An experimental investigation of the possible anti-social use of hypnosis."

The word 'possible' in the second title gives you a flavour of how that experiment was conducted and the intent behind it.

The two experiments were conducted almost identically with the hypnotist suggesting that harm may be caused to the experimenter by the volunteer subjects.

Delivering Suggestion

I used to believe that there are particular ways and formats to deliver suggestion, to the point where, until recently, I gave out rules for suggestion on courses.

Hey, we all make mistakes.

In fact it doesn't matter how you put a suggestion together providing it makes sense to the respondents' subconscious mind, and that it can model and make use of your suggestion.

There is an established theory that states you shouldn't mention the object of the problem as that will make the mind think about it. Yes, that's right; this wonderful school of thought says that you shouldn't get the mind to think about smoking if you want it to stop smoking. It doesn't take much thought to realise that doing one without the other is actually impossible.

For instance I used to tell students what I was taught, to only use phrases such as "Free from tobacco", "no longer needing to put inappropriate substances in your body" and other such things.

If you are one of those guys then I apologise. I was being a therapist.

What I do now is much more direct and akin to suggestion delivery on stage. If I want them to stop smoking I tell them they don't smoke. I'll say that smoking isn't part of their lives and that it doesn't affect them. They don't have cravings because non-smokers don't have cravings and they won't be tempted to smoke because they are a non-smoker and don't smoke.

If they want to get rid of a phobia I tell them not to be scared of X because they aren't, never have been and never will be.

If I feel it necessary I will also use symbolism to fasten this behaviour of thinking although the above can work just as well without it in 90% of cases.

Keep suggestions simple and direct.

Deliver it in a matter of fact way, as if it was already their, and your, reality.

Say, "You don't smoke", not "you no longer smoke" or "you will not smoke".

Use your, and their, everyday language.

If it's not comfortable for you don't ramble on about being able to remain passive and in control in times of social discord – that's from a script I just read from the internet – instead try using what you would in a normal conversation.

"You can stay calm even when others are getting up your nose. It doesn't bother you. You just chill."

Go into your imagination and feel the emotions you want them to feel, so that your delivery will be full of that.

If a suggestion doesn't work immediately don't repeat it. Rephrase it.

Let's look at the old myth of suggestions being rejected.

In all of the books I've read on the subject of hypnosis the rejection of suggestion is always put forward as if it were rule and law. I think this came about in this way.

A hypnotist sometime gave someone who was apparently hypnotised a suggestion. The hypnotee did not react to the suggestion. And so it was observed that the hypnotee must **A**: Be in control of some kind of reasoning process, and **B**: Be able to decide whether to accept or reject the suggestion.

Let's look at the other possibilities, we'll ignore the obvious one that the person may not have been hypnotised at all.

A: The hypnotee didn't understand what the suggestion was meant to make them do, **B**: The hypnotee had no internal model on which to base a response.

How often does the average hypnotherapist check to see if the person they are working with understands the suggestion? On average I'd guess at never during the process and hardly ever afterwards. It beggars belief that it's not standard procedure to make sure they understand what you are telling them to do. This is especially true if you've decided to use a metaphor without backing up with direct suggestion.

The amazing thing is that it is so easy to check. I do this all the time, after saying something to them I ask them to nod their head if they understand. I don't use complex ideo-motor responses or IMR's which you may have read about; such as telling them to lift a finger when their subconscious is in agreement because when they do lift it they may just be responding to the suggestion and not agreeing at all. No, let's keep it direct and simple - a nod is an ideo-motor response. It isn't something we generally do consciously and it's almost hard wired in as the affirmative in the western world. So ask if they understand.

Next word the suggestion so that it fits their sphere of probable understanding. It's no good suggesting that they will see themselves doing something if they have no idea of how that would go.

I was once doing a show for adults during which I did a striptease routine with the men on stage. I only ever allowed shirts and tops to come off – that was horrible enough at times – and put the suggestion in by telling them that they were the 'Full Monty' from the film and book of the same name.

On this one occasion one gentleman didn't join the others when the sounds of Tom Jones singing Kiss blasted through the room and he just stood there looking confused. To an outside observer, especially one who believed that suggestions could be rejected, it would have been easy to assume that the guy found the suggestion distasteful and had rejected it.

For me at the time that wasn't an option. I went up to the guy and off mic asked if he knew who the Full Monty were. He shrugged and shook his head. It turned out afterward that he was a school teacher from South Africa and hadn't seen the film or read the book.

So, he had no model of experience on which to base his reaction. Not even one of observation or even one that had been installed by anecdote. I noticed though that he was wearing a wedding ring and re-induced him telling him he was at home doing a sexy striptease for his partner in time to the music and guess what – the best strip I ever saw.

A hypnotised person can not reject suggestion if they understand it and can base their reaction and use of that on some inner model. If a suggestion doesn't work therefore it is down to the fact that the hypnotist didn't do it right.

Always check they understand and don't make a suggestion so airy and confusing that only you and some bloke on top of a mountain in Outer Mongolia could understand it.

KEEP IT SIMPLE

The ʃuper ʃuggestion

Again this is another cross over from the stage book. This is really the only 'suggestion' you need. After this you can stop 'suggesting' and just tell them to stop.

Goes like this,

"From this moment in time every word I say instantly becomes your reality."

If you don't get that then don't use it. Basically what it means is that the hypnotee will experience what the hypnotist tells them to experience, will believe what the hypnotist tells them to believe and will know what the hypnotist tells them they will know.

Maybe ultimate suggestion would be better than super.

Vocal Tones

How important are vocal tones?

Now I've seen lots of people suggest that these are not important however I know that although I'm speaking more or less normally in phrasing and accent, I also know I speak in a certain way when I'm hypnotising. What my partner Jane calls my 'hypnotic voice', and always have.

In fact every good hypnotist I have ever watched work does this.

Without doubt the intent of the hypnotist is more important than the willingness or co-operation of the hypnotee. And the most obvious way that the hypnotee picks this up when we are working closed eyes is through the voice. Because of this it's good to understand the importance of vocal tones.

By vocal tones I mean pacing and intonation. Not whether you should go up or down at the end. Roll your 'r's or put some vibrato at the end. No, I am talking about the cadence, the rhythm and perhaps the lilt of your voice.

With singers the tone reflects the focus the performer has on the content of the song. In hypnosis the tone reflects the focus the hypnotist has on the intent of the suggestion.

If you feel warbling fits the bill best, and for you it works wonderfully well, it isn't working so fantastically because this is the definitive way to deliver a suggestion, or that this is better for the recipient. It's working because it's the best thing for you.

For instance I know one thing for a fact, it's easier to hypnotise a group of people whilst being amplified through a PA and speaker system than it is doing it dry.

That's because what's being amplified is the tone and intonation. The intent.

So, when you are delivering suggestions, what can aid them being accepted is to use your 'Hypnotists voice'. That is your way of speaking which immediately feels comfortable for you and which also feels the most focused.

There is a school of thought that lowering your voice, or talking in a monotone way is soporific and therefore hypnotic. It isn't.

There is another school that thinks that pausing at inappropriate times such as Erickson used to, is hypnotic, it isn't. I rather think that Erickson paused because after two polio attacks his diaphragm was shot and pausing in the middle of a sentence to actually breath was a no choice thing.

There is a school of thought when recording so called hypnotic audio that two voices, one on each track is hypnotic. It is not.

However there is an anomaly here because guess what? All of the above can aid hypnosis even though none of them is necessary for hypnosis.

Again though, this isn't about the vocal tones or clever speech patterns, it is about your intent and your beliefs and behaviours.

If any of the above is necessary for you to feel comfortable and capable as a hypnotist then it's your intent that gives them their power.

I'm told my voice changes when I turn the hypnosis on and I guess it does. However I think that is more to do with people tuning in to my intent rather than any particular change in tone. There certainly is nothing deliberate going on.

So, unless you feel differently there is no need to bother about developing any particular vocal tones, just talk.

There is no doubt that pausing occasionally and allowing the hypnotee to process what you said is a good move but it really doesn't seem to matter when or where you do this. I do think it makes your voice sound different and adds a touch of mystery which appeals to the mind.

The fact is there is no consistency in reports of whether this is more or less effective. I think it's entirely down to the operator to decide which way to work and the important thing is that you work comfortably.

The obvious thing is most of the time your voice is your number one tool and you should really look after it. Never let your throat dry while working and always work with a glass of water to hand. Never consume dairy produce or chocolate before working as these increase mucus production.

Finally remember that your voice is a muscle, if you don't use it you'll lose it. Exercise your voice. Singing is by far the best way to do this, it's fun and annoys the hell out of your family, friends and neighbours.

Anchors And Post Hypnotic Suggestion

Anchoring or post hypnotic is the way you ensure that whatever pattern you have installed in the clients reality is confirmed regularly and has less chance of being overridden by the other hypnotists in their life such as family, peer groups and colleges.

Remember everyone is a hypnotist and if you don't anchor your work in some way or suggest that the new pattern will not be overridden by anyone else, then even though your work was a complete success it could be that in a month or so your client is back to square one and no better off than they were before.

To ensure longevity then we anchor or rather attach the pattern of belief or behaviour to another belief, behaviour or action.

One of the most common anchors usually taught in hypnotherapy schools comes from the thought that making something conscious and deliberate ensures its success. So the client is told to touch their finger and thumb together every time they want or need to fire the anchor. They are told this after the hypnosis and it is rarely installed during the session.

I can't see why people think this will work.

In my experience such anchors are rarely used and are soon forgotten. Basically when people come to a hypnotist they can't or don't want to actively change their behaviours, they want you to do it. So giving them home work isn't what they pay for.

Okay so this isn't empowering them – that's what Chinosis is for – but it is the way things really are at least some of the time.

So, if we are not going to trust that they will use a deliberate anchor how can we establish anchors for them? Simple, we associate desired action or behaviour, but more importantly needed beliefs and emotions to anything we know that will without doubt happen.

Why use anything but the predictable when the average day for most people is stuffed full of non-emotive events which can be used to anchor new patterns to.

From putting their feet on the floor at the start of their day through brushing their teeth, combing their hair, dressing, opening a door, having breakfast – through to brushing their teeth and going to bed the world is full of natural actions to which we can anchor.

A simple post hypnotic anchor such as, "And every time you open a door that feeling of confidence and self worth grows and glows through every pore and fibre of your mind and body making you feel that wonderful glow of energy and calm..." will result in around twenty or thirty firings of that anchor a day. It will work on every door. Bedroom, bathroom, kitchen, Front door, car door, office, workshop, shop, store... and that really is just a beginning.

So anchor **simply** and **easily** to anything you are sure will happen and, preferably, that is unlikely to hold an emotive pattern in itself.

A final note. Not all apparent post hypnotics are that. When you see a hypnotist working on stage and they say, "One two wide awake." Then subjects respond to the suggestion, they are in fact still in hypnosis. They have to be as it were 'released' from the state before the reaction becomes post hypnotic.

That is they have to be formally told the hypnosis is finished.

There is also what could be considered to be something of a hypnotic hangover. Even when the session is ended and for some minutes after the hypnotee is still in a state where suggestion is readily accepted even to the degree of when formally and completely hypnotised.

This can be very useful. A lot of good work can be done in the conversation directly following the session.

"That was a brilliant session. One of the best ever. Did you notice when you said - or did XXX?"

I've even used this time to do something I'd forgotten or had thought of too late. And of course I always use it to give more feel good suggestions.

∫criptnotism

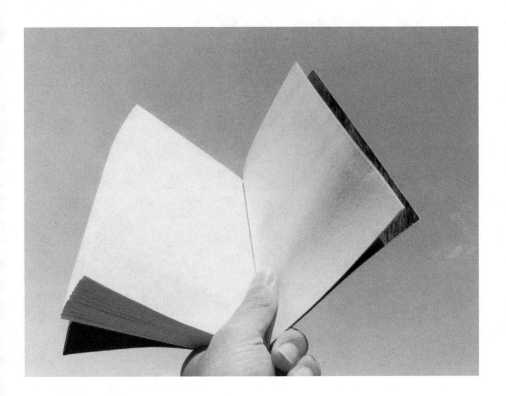

I'm often asked why I don't make a point of supplying loads of scripts to people who attend at seminars and courses; well there are good reasons for this.

No script is effective.

Hypnotists are effective.

It's like the bits of paper we give out at the end of courses. No one get hypnotised by a qualification, they get hypnotised by a hypnotist.

I suppose scripts are okay for getting some inspiration or if you are doing a stage presentation the trouble with scripts though is that if you have to think about getting it word perfect you won't do the job as effectively. Your intent is not focused on the hypnotee or the hypnosis but on the script itself.

If you do believe that scripts can help you formulate your own approaches then when you read a script look at the intent behind it. Go for getting its feel and understanding its target. The owner of the script probably found it very useful to them in the situation it came to them, but sadly that isn't usually the case. The majority of scripts are written cold and with no intention at all and sadly often no practise, making them as useful as a chocolate teapot.

I always smile when I read that scripts can help with this exact type of therapy or hypnotee. If there is any benefit from purchasing and reading a script it's the author who benefits, not the hypnotee or hypnotist.

In practice few people can actually remember them and I have seen lots of people reading them to hypnotees on courses I have attended but have seen very little hypnosis going on there.

They would probably have had as much chance of inducing scriptnosis if they hit the hypnotee with the script than they would reading it verbatim to them.

Your voice is not natural when you're reading unless you are an extremely good actor. Then again good actors don't read. They recite and interpret. Rustling bits of paper won't help either. The mind might be the intellectual equivalent of a bright nine-year-old, however a nine-year-old isn't stupid and can usually recognise incompetence, and might just wonder why you need the bits of paper. And remember that the hypnotee's mind is entirely, completely and absolutely concentrated on the hypnotist, on you and what you are doing. So any hesitation or doubt will be picked up and acted upon just the same as saying "Don't trust me, this isn't true."

I've nothing against people reading scripts for inspiration before they're actually working with someone, but please put them away and become a hypnotist not a scriptnotist.

For that reason in this book we've included the odd phrase and our Hypnosology head and except for the wake up script these words and phrases should be considered nothing more than **backbones,** which, although they don't give a word for word lyric, they will give you a basis upon which you can build for some varying techniques.

We have found this to be the best way to encourage your creativity. And it's creativity which I feel is the difference between a bloody good hypnotist and somebody who just talks at people.

Hypnotic or
ʃeventh ʃense

Some people just know the right thing to say. Everyone knows them. They may be a colleague, a friend, a bar-person, a teacher, your boss or the family oldie.

They are the ones whose advice is nearly always spot on, if only sometimes taken on board and carried through.

They are the ones people gravitate towards in times of adversity. The ones who, without asking a question more probing than "How are you?", are immediately inundated by the complete and unabridged life story of the person they asked.

They are also the ones who listen to all that and don't judge. But they do feel what is right and productive for all concerned.

They are often the people who gravitate towards arts such as hypnosis because that feels right as well.

This intuitive and innate skill is often called the sixth sense of which apparently only a certain proportion of the population are lucky enough to have. I don't think that's the case at all. I think that everyone has a sixth sense but some people have a seventh.

I think that when knowing what to do in hypnosis we do indeed tap into a 'sense' which tells us which approach and which techniques to use for the best. I think that everyone has the potential for this and that it is indeed natural, but as with many innate skills it is dimmed and dulled by the way we are dragged up through childhood and, educationally and socially, imaginatively castrated.

Many natural abilities are concealed because overriding social belief patterns are installed; fortunately all we need do is tune into them and change our patterns. All we need do is begin to trust and listen to our inner voices and follow their lead. Or ideally just allow instinct to use us and shrug off our limiting learning.

To do this let's use the seventh or hypnotic sense. Maybe I'm being poetic, but I do rather like to think that there *is* a further sense, and the best hypnotists I have ever seen have all had a well developed hypnotic sense. The most effective all work far more by instinct in the moment than by logic or planning. By sense rather than sentence.

Developing any of your senses is easily achieved, by using them, by becoming aware of them, and learning to trust them to the point where you can ignore them again.

The hypnotic sense tells you when hypnosis is in place. It tells you when to start and when to end. It's this sense that will also tell you how things are going inside the hypnotee's reality when not a lot is happening on the outside. Trust it.

Let it take you into the moment and join the hypnotee in their reality. You'll know what and where that is, you will. Just don't intellectualise any of this. That's like trying to make sense and logic out of sex which, at best, is a smelly and altogether too physical a pursuit, but amazingly good fun when you roll with it.

The channel of communication which is hypnosis is a two-way path and without doubt you can very easily tune into your internal terminal and listen in to theirs.

Call it instinct. Call it guessing. Call it precognition. Call it telepathy. Call it 'Thalmic Communication'. Call it Fred, which is as good a name as any.

It doesn't matter, it does happen. The lack of a suitable label or of any scientific explanation doesn't stop it working; only you can do that by looking for it too hard. It doesn't work in any logical sense, and you will never actually find it, so just forget it and tune in.

This is one of those points that unfortunately you will never get from a book, DVD or audio. This is one of those things that just has to be experienced and it is the experience that makes the difference. Don't let this stop you experimenting as it really is a natural thing and you do have it.

Pacing

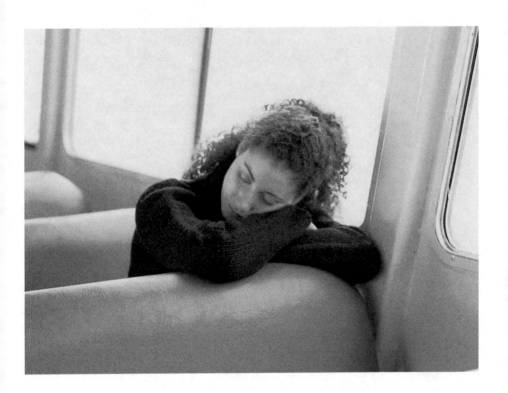

As with the rest of the stuff in this book, this understanding of pacing is mine. It isn't a rule. And like lots of other things, you can get this wrong and still get hypnosis. The thing is that when you get this right, it will increase the accuracy of your inductive phase and raise your success rate no end.

A lot has been said in endless books about ways of building rapport and matching other people. And as we've already said most of these really only work in theory, or when it's happened anyway, or just in the seminar room where everyone knows the score and what is expected of them. And with a charismatic presenter, Awe rapport happens.

I recently read a book, just one of umpteen thousand that all report this rubbish, telling me that everyone used a speech pattern which showed how they were centred and focused. A visual person for instance will use visual language such as 'see', 'sight' and will pepper their speech with colours and visual descriptions.

An auditory person will use sound words and will 'hear' what you are saying; a kinetic person will 'touch' ground with you and 'feel' what you are saying.

It's great as a theory until you get someone who says, "You know I really feel right about the way I see this. Sounds like your taste is smooth." Which slightly screws you up on the calibration, or you just get the person who says next to nothing apart from no and yes, so you've lost yet another 'matching' tool.

My understanding of pacing however, is not to match the dominant patterns people exhibit but to take account of something much more enlightening, and to apply it to pace as in racing and take note of the speed at which the hypnotees do what they do.

131

Different people work at different speeds and at different times. Those of you who have seen stage hypnosis at work will doubtless have noticed how the stage may be full of volunteers at the start, and only have a handful left at the end. The main factor at play here is speed and nothing more.

The stage performer doesn't have the time to notice how fast or slowly people are reacting to their suggestions. And unless the performer is really boring, and takes 40 minutes before they begin the first routine and are able to slow down, they will work with, and indeed only work with, those who are paced at the fast end of rapid at that particular time.

It has *nothing* to do with how suggestible someone is and *everything* to do with how fast they are working internally.

It is pacing that helps maintain and manage the state. Slow stage hypnotists may get more volunteers induced, but will lose more during the show as they have to speed up to prevent the thing becoming boring. Fast performers may start with fewer, but on the whole have closer to that number at the curtain because there is less change in the speed of delivery.

If the majority of the people on stage are working at the fastest speed imaginable then they will be unable to speed up and will not slow down so they remain fairly consistent.

Of course the advantage of consultation in one-to-one situations, or even in group work where the situation is more intimate or less fear invoking than on a comedy stage, is that there is time to pace your delivery and speed of working to theirs initially and, as they speed up, get them to a position where you are leading the pace and they are following you.

This is hard to explain without seeing it but try this… pick someone to approach across a room at a party, in an office, shop wherever, and notice their breathing. Don't stare too hard even if their back is toward you because they will pick this up and look your way – if you don't believe that try it.

Now if they are breathing slowly and deeply, walk slowly up to them and introduce yourself. Use the old do I know you approach. You will notice that their whole demeanour will match their breathing. People resonate at a pace which goes through everything. A slower person will even blink more slowly and languidly. A fast person will blink rapidly and often.

In a consultation setting it is very easy to observe someone's pace. If you have personally talked to them, even on the telephone, you will already have an idea of what this is. But on meeting you will get a fuller impression. Slow people will speak low and slow, they will pause and reflect before answering questions, and will give your hand a squeeze rather than a shake.

Fast people will have their life story out before they sit down and dislocate an elbow to show how pleased they are to meet you. The average person will be somewhere in the middle of this. But it is my observation that average is not normal and most of the time people are one or the other. There are lots of turtles and hares but only a few 'Turtares'.

In consultation hypnotic terms, there are usually far more hares. People seem to speed up as a defence mechanism. It's no good being slow if you think you may have to duck to avoid ballistic suggestions. So choosing to be thinking and behaving faster is the predictable result of fear. The good old flight or fight thingy which apparently causes stress. For that reason and the fact that a lot of people still slightly fear the hypnotist the majority are more successful at rapid inductions than they are at slow.

As I explained in rapport, people like people who like them, and are more inclined to resonate with someone they like or respect. This is also true of the pace which they are inclined towards. The evidence of the stage hypnotist shows that slower-inclined people will not respond to rapidly-inclined approaches by the hypnotist. And the failure of those trained in progressive and slow relaxation methods reflects that fast people don't respond to the slow approach. For that reason it's the slow relaxotherapist who has the problem of getting rid of fear before they can work. A rapid hypnotist will just use the fear and the fast pace required to zonk the faster thinking hypnotee, and will be able to easily slow a little to affect the slower paced.

So all you need do is to pace to them. At first.

If they are slow then slowly build towards your induction, if fast just go for it. Although by slow I mean taking a couple of minutes rather than a few seconds.

During your induction phase slow down if they are a slow paced person, speed up if they are fast. Watch for the minute, and for the massive changes. We can sometimes miss a change in deep breathing because we are waiting for REM.

Use these points of change, such as taking a deep swallow or breath, stopping or starting of REM, a shift in muscle rigidity or flaccidness, or even a smile, as indicators for you moving things along.

Use these changes in pacing as a signal to tell the hypnotee how well things are going, using the old Erickson phrase of "That's right" no matter what is happening. If there is a change say, "That's right".

The remarkable thing about pacing is that the more the hypnotee is taken in and out of the state, the more competent, or the more easily established the communication becomes, the faster the pace becomes for both of you.

In my experience it is important that the pace quickens. As I said some people start more slowly but speed up, however a fast person does not slow down. Familiarity with the state always causes things to go faster. Just think how riding a bicycle goes from wobbling at two miles an hour to free wheeling at twenty. How a stumbling toddle in kindergarten becomes a graceful gallop across a school playing field.

As we get used to things, we speed up. As we grow in confidence and competence, we speed up. Even the slowest person will eventually be easily as fast as the naturally fastest after just a few moments of experiencing the state of hypnosis. They become easier and then faster to induce. Faster to respond and to influence. So the more they get induced, the better they become at being hypnotised, and the faster their response time becomes.

It's important you watch and understand this because the better they become, the faster you have to work as well. If you don't match this acceleration and keep up, then an awful lot of the time you will lose them as they get tired of waiting for you.

I think that it's pacing that has led to the myth that the hypnotised can leave the state when they decide to do so. I've not seen that. But I have in trials observed that my speed, when it's not matched with theirs, seems to cause a confusion which is enough to lose the mind's dominance and bring them back to their previous state.

ʃtate Management

Once you've got hypnosis, the most important part of the process now comes into play, that of maintaining and managing the state.

Most of the time, if you are pacing right and working quickly, you'll find that the hypnotee manages to stay in this place with no effort from the hypnotist. But you are human and that means you can, and will, need to keep things as you need them to be.

Emotional states and moods change all the time. If the hypnotist doesn't watch that then this could easily lead to the old misapprehension that the hypnotees can decide to open their eyes at any time and walk away. This is wrong, simply because it presumes that the **hypnotee** has a choice, not that the hypnotist has been negligent in observing whether the state is being maintained or not.

In my opinion what has led to this myth is that **the hypnotist is not in control** of the situation. Just as with any other mental state, if the point of focus here is removed or diluted in anyway, we find that the mind will drift and wonder, and I do mean wonder. Wonder what the hell is going on.

So if the hypnotist doesn't maintain the strength and focus of the hypnotic connection, continuously keep tuning and refreshing the state, then things will return back to where they were before.

Just like a rubber band, the mind can be stretched any which way. But, let it go, and it will always return to it's state of stasis. It can be stretched into the hypnotic state, but it sure as hell won't stay there forever.

However, providing the hypnotist doesn't allow control to go back into its neutral state, then the situation remains entirely in the hands of the operator, the band remains stretched, and you can work.

Maintaining and managing the state is very easy to do. Continuous reminders to the subconscious of what the expectations and intents are and regular checks and tests of the acceptance of suggestibility are easily put into place.

By far the easiest way of doing this is to give them something to do that will continue throughout the session. For instance getting a hand to float in midair and just leaving it there, watch for the hand dropping even minutely. When it does, just suggest that it's regaining its altitude.

Give them a command word and suggest that they smile every time it's spoken. Make it an unusual word; I use the word Cherokee as did one of my teachers. It may be common in the United States, but you don't get many Cherokees on the English Rivera in Devon, so I find it a safe and handy word to use. It should be obvious that all you then have to do is drop the word Cherokee into the conversation as much as possible and watch the reaction. Tell them that the word will take them into an even deeper and more intense state and it becomes doubly useful.

By far and away, the easiest and simplest way to make maintaining the hypnotic state easy, is to keep the actual hypnosis sessions, that is the trance states, as short as possible. Don't think that your hypnotee needs to be hypnotised the whole 50 minutes if they have booked an hour session. It is usually far more productive to have them hypnotised four times in six or seven minute sessions.

Using each re-induction to fine tune and intensify your hypnotic connection.

Working in this way means that you don't have to concentrate through periods longer than the average. I've never figured out why the hypnotist is supposed to be better at concentrating like this than the average person, I certainly am not. Remember, you are only human.

The small breaks also alert you to anything untoward that may be happening to the hypnotee such as a numb backside or an encroaching toilet break. It also allows you to test how successful your suggestions have been.

This leads quite naturally on to the next section where you will see that, even though I say here 'hypnotised for a few minutes', we never actually bring them out of it.

Wide Awake Hypnosis

It would be absolutely true to say that all hypnosis is waking hypnosis. Hypnosis is not sleep.

In saying that, waking hypnosis has become a recognised, separate way of working in as much as the hypnotee's eyes are open, their apparent cognitive capacity is normal, and they answer questions as if nothing were untowardly different from their average state of mind. At the same time the little finger is still stuck in their right ear and they can't remember their name.

Any stage hypnotist will tell you that this is how most hypnosis works anyway. The sleep, relaxation, and nodding heads are all part of the show, not part of the hypnosis. By waking hypnosis, what we actually mean is the acceptance of suggestion without a discernible trance state. This is, of course, what happens naturally when we are accepting suggestions. We are wide awake.

"Go down here, turn right, go past the old football pitch, down to the Dirty Duck pub, turn right again and there you are."

That isn't a suggestion, it is a direction. But if the person wants to go where we are telling them to go, they will accept that direction and go there. Or just decide to go to a different restaurant. Wide awake hypnosis works differently because the choice isn't in place at all.

I have often said the following and had it work supremely well with no other setup than the fact that I'm a hypnotist and my intent is in place and so I am being believed.

Do this at an entirely inappropriate point in general conversation. It's what NLPers apparently call a pattern interrupt. I call it a suggestion because that is what it was before NLP, and calling something by another name doesn't change it.

So in an offhand, but quite determined way, pick your target and say,
"Have you noticed that you can't put your hand on your knee? There seems to be some kind of force field that's stopping you from doing that, that's interesting isn't it?"

Now that's a suggestion. And if the person's subconscious mind really wants to go there and experience it, then they will, regardless of what the conscious mind thinks about it, and regardless of whether they are 'hypnotised' or not.

I can't state this strongly enough. The difference between the two is that in the first case the conscious mind wanted to go there. In the second the subconscious, or mind, wanted to go there. In the first there was choice; that is the conscious mind had a choice, in the second there was acceptance and, once accepted, the conscious mind can no longer choose. If the conscious mind can choose, then we have no hypnosis.

When this happens naturally in the course of our lives it is always waking hypnosis. If at a time when your mind is dominant somebody suggests to it that you are less than good in some way, maybe they say you are ugly, useless, boring, or just a plain waste of space; if that is accepted and implemented by your mind, then that is waking hypnosis.

So, giving a suggestion to somebody when they are not obviously in a hypnotic trance in such a way that the suggestion is accepted can be called waking or wide awake hypnosis.

This should not be mistaken as NLP, although this state of affairs is usually the only time that the practice of what a friend of mine calls Nauseatingly Lengthy Pantomime actually works—when it **is** hypnosis.

Such things work because the intent is to make the mind dominant **or** to make use of the fact that it is. **In hypnosis intent is everything.**

The 'BUZZ'
ſafe 'Wakeup' Procedure

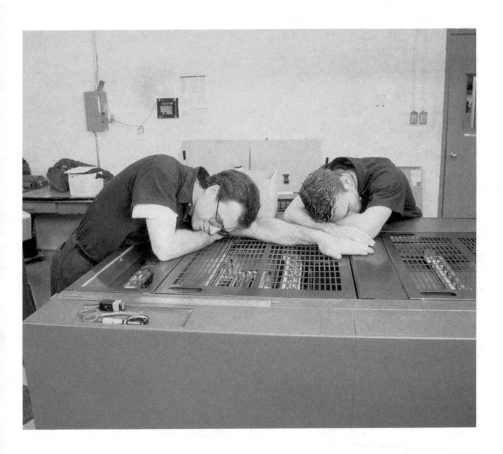

One of the most important things in any ritualised hypnosis session is that both the hypnotist and hypnotee know when it is over.

This may seem obvious but mostly isn't. You could get away with just saying, "One two, back to normal!" after putting in one or two suggestions of feeling wide awake and normal. However, being very much a practical and professional person, I always think that there are one or two things that should be considered.

The first being that the hypnotee is absolutely chock-full of suggestions, belief patterns, and all sorts of rubbish picked up along their life's highway which you know nothing about. This **could** include the belief that hypnosis gives you a headache, spots, bubonic plague, and makes your hair fall out.

They won't know they have this baggage on board, and neither will you. So treat it like driving at night after the bars have turned out. Just assume that everyone else on the road is drunk – including you – and take some extra care.

I've always thought that it is very important to clear out anything that may stop them feeling anything but wonderful before it's had chance to kick in. So, having picked up this wake-up procedure, and I've no idea where from, I know it so well I could say it in my sleep, and I've used it exclusively for a long time.

The important thing in a successful hypnosis session, and possibly the *most* important, is that they come out of hypnosis feeling wonderful. No matter how good, bad, or indifferent the actual session was, there is no doubt that if they feel amazing physically and mentally at the end of it this goes a long way to convince the mind that the process was successful. Very often this can even make the difference between success and failure.

I know I don't like scripts but the following is the one I've used for over 30 years and it's never let me down. I believe that it originated on the stage as have most of the more productive techniques involved in hypnosis. I'll give you the script first and then I will break it down into its constituents and have a look at them.

Wake up Script

"In a moment I'm going to bring you back to full awareness. I'll count from one to five and on the number five you will open your eyes and stretch, feeling completely refreshed and alive. It's like you've had eight hours sleep. However, being hypnotised is not sleep and when you next go to bed you will sleep better than you have for years and awake at the appropriate time feeling refreshed and revitalized, just as you will when I get to the number five.

"So, one!
Every nerve, every muscle becoming fully awake and fully aware.

"Two:
Feel that huge surge of energy go right through your body.

"Three:
Take a deep, deep breath of cool, clear, mountain air, filling your lungs and feeling that energy-giving oxygen going through every nerve, muscle and fibre.

"Four: you can feel that cool, clear, mountain water washing through your head, your chest, your body. Your stomach and chest are clear. Your head is clear. Your throat and nose are clear. Your eyes are bright and shiny and...

[Clap your hands loudly] "Five! WIDE AWAKE! And stretch..."

Make every word a direct command. Lift your voice as you go through the numbers and emphasise the emotive words and action words such as 'clear', 'energy', and 'bright and shiny'. Make them fill their lungs and stretch.

It could be argued that all of the above was unnecessary if you have somebody truly hypnotised, then just saying open your eyes is enough. But we're talking here about ritualised hypnosis, and the ritual goes all the way through. Not only that, this gives an amazing physical 'buzz' to the hypnotee.

The important thing, more than anything else, is the oxygenation of the body. The suggestions of energy certainly work and I've often seen people report that they felt a tingle in their fingers and toes. Getting oxygen into them will have exactly this effect, especially if you been in there for a while and they haven't moved much. A deep breath coupled with stretching always makes you feel good, try it right now and see what I mean.

On the number four we negate any sluggish after-effects while at the same time overriding any suggestions that may hold that hypnosis causes headaches or leaves you feeling bunged up or mucus full.

You don't have to use this word for word but it is important that you get the general feel right and do the oxygenation!

I also clap just as I say wide awake, it makes them jump and gives them a little rush of adrenalin, which helps produce The Hypnotic Buzz, which is the last thing they'll experience and therefore the first thing they'll remember when they go home and talk about the session with others.

Just to add the cherry on the cake, I always smile and sit up straight as the first thing I want them to see as they leave the state is a happy, smiling and confident hypnotist.

It also helps if you stretch and breath deeply with them. This goes a long way to get you out of hypnotist mode and back into the wide awake and alert person you need to be.

I always feel that the best sessions are the ones where I don't always remember what happened. It's the hypnotic connection thing I guess.

Maybe we even become a little hypnotised ourselves. I think we do and should.

So waking them should also be waking you and you should get the hypnotic buzz as well.

Finally remember the old adage that bad news gets twice around the world before good news has got its boots on.

Send a soporific and sluggish client out of your office and how many of their friends will come see you?

Send a bouncing happy energy ball out and just try stopping them coming.

Hypnotic Symbolism

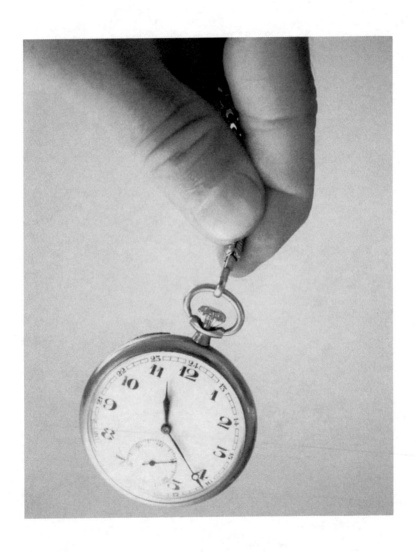

Using hypnotic symbolism has changed the way I work entirely. Although I will use direct suggestion on things like smoking not everything is so clear cut. Often people don't know what's wrong and, even though I am a good guesser, I don't feel right about guessing what that might be for them.

While working on the non-relaxation, non-trance form of energy based self help we call Chinosis, I came to thinking about how we use patterns in our mind. How we symbolise stuff. Symbolism has simplified everything and is what I use for everything, even if only to concrete the work in place.

I've always had a fairly good success rate, but now it's through the roof. Symbolism makes things happen faster, easier, and in my experience far more comfortably for the hypnotee, especially when the consultation involves having to deal with long-standing issues.

So what is hypnotic symbolism?

Symbolism – is the language our mind uses. The inner mind thinks and communicates in patterns and shapes, in impressions, emotions and feelings. Our conscious interprets these and uses words to describe these patterns, both to itself and the outside world. Hypnotic symbolism is using the originating symbol, rather than the interpreted words, deliberately, as the way of directly communicating with and the focusing of the mind.

Symbolism is how we talk – to ourselves – or rather the way our illogical mind talks to our reasoning and logical brain. Neither speaks the same 'language' as such. So I think it's important that the hypnotist learns to 'speak' to them in the language that they understand.

In the past, in hypnosis, the symbolism or visualisation used has usually been given, or at least guided, by the hypnotist. In Hypnotic Symbolism we ask the hypnotee to get what's there and do not consciously attempt to control or analyse the symbols that come forward. In this way we avoid impressing our own preconceived conscious assumptions on the situation and stop those of the hypnotee being used also.

The symbols used in Hypnotic Symbolism should 'only' come from the client, and then only from their mind, not their conscious brain. The hypnotist should be especially careful not to lead here. Absolutely not. Never. I usually ask them to close their eyes (so that nothing in the room will impose a symbol) but that's all. Usually symbols are interpreted as being visual but it's vital that the hypnotist doesn't impose this. Symbols can be anything. Pictures, feelings, smells, sounds, or just the feelings that emotions produce. Butterflies in the stomach are a good example of this.

Hypnotic Symbolism is unique to the individual. One of the more interesting things I do in seminars and classes is to ask three or four people to obtain their symbol for childhood. Not one will ever be the same – ever. Our internal symbolism is exceptional and distinct. And with this technique the hypnotist does not need to know what that is. I don't ask what their symbol is in consultation, and if told, I smile and say "Really? Okay let's work with that..." You must **not** interpret; you must **not** presume you understand the meaning of a blob of green slime. In short you must not, no matter how intuitive or educated it may be, **guess an interpretation of the symbol.**

I believe that one of the greatest problems in cognitive therapies is being told by another, what X means. For instance, I once had a guy who was working on his weight tell me his symbol was a balloon. Right, applying logic seems pretty straight forward – balloon – round – circular – inflated. However he smiled and when I asked if he felt any of these things applied his reply was, "Good lord no. It's parties. Always stuff myself stupid at parties, at Christmas...."

The balloon to 'him', that is to his brain, represented a place and time, not his physical shape. But, what if it actually represented something else? We couldn't know, could we? Not for sure. Only his mind really knows.

I had to admit I could have been wrong there, and so could he. We held different patterns. Different symbols. We spoke the same language, but in an entirely different way. I think I'm not far off when I say the reason therapies have a failure rate is because of this lack of accuracy in our communication.

We know misdiagnosis happens a lot in the established medical world. I have direct experience of this when I was told that my neuro-muscular condition was 'Frederic's Ataxia' – a condition which with luck lets you live till forty or so. In fact I have Charcott Marie Tooth syndrome which, although bothersome, does not lead to early termination. I spent a couple of very depressed years until being re-diagnosed, virtually waiting to die, all because someone was wrong in interpretation and diagnosis. That will not happen with my people, and hopefully it won't happen with yours.

So, don't diagnose or guess or assume that because the client appears to have X then the cause could be Y. You may be right 80% of the time, but just as easily you could be wrong by the same margin. You owe it to your clients, and just as importantly to yourself, not to risk failure because you were wrong. Think of it this way, you know how the car works because you know what is under the bonnet, but you don't know what's in the glove-box and that may be more important.

That is the beauty of Hypnotic Symbolism, it simply takes out any chance of operator error. All symbols are abstract. This is the hardest thing you have to get over to the client, and the hardest thing you have to understand yourself. Symbols are subjective. Don't try to make sense of it.

If you have a fear of spiders, your inner mind may give you the image of a window or a flower pot. It might just as happily give you a hairy daffodil or an elevator. It is vital that you don't consciously expect that this should be the image of the spider or maybe a web.

JUST GO WITH WHATEVER THE MIND GIVES YOU— NO MATTER WHAT.

It is very easy to get caught in what we think the thing should be, and spend way too much time being clever, and second guessing our clients' needs, instead of listening. Making sense of the inner mind is a huge and usually thankless task because if the mind were logical and made sense then there would be no need for a conscious logical filter. We would not have emotions and emotional clutter, and life would be hellishly boring and without excitement, thrill, beauty or meaning.

It's also easy to forget that, although we human beings communicate most of the time using words, the mind sees these as it does everything else, as patterns and symbols. For instance, we SAY "cat", and, as a result of its symbol-matching system, the mind gives us the mental image of a small playful bundle of furry delight… or the image of half a ton of striped eating machine, with human on the menu, or a razor blade.

For now, think of the language of symbolism as a British person talking to an American with the common language of English. The basic words are understood, but the subtleties of meaning can be missed thanks to one of the versions being wrong and using words in an unfortunate way, often leading to confusion and misinterpretation.

In our communication with the outside world, it is our conscious mind that is dominant for most of the time. It acts, as I've said, like a filter, apparently allowing what is useful to 'sink in' or 'come out' and rejecting the rest. However, there are times when this protective filter can be by-passed and the inner mind communicated with directly, as in hypnosis.

All these things are direct communication from the inner mind, which is why, under logical analysis, they often make little or no sense. To make sense we need to analyse them, and during that analysis, which is the process of translation by the conscious mind, there is the problem of not knowing enough words of the common language to effect an accurate translation. However, with just a little guidance, it is possible to achieve this communication, and focus it, so that it is very accurate indeed.

The symbol for the issue we wish to address could be anything; a visual pattern such as a face, an object or even a colour. It could just as easily be a sensory pattern; a smell, a tune, a taste or a touch. It's important that the hypnotee understands that **a symbol could be anything at all**, make this absolutely clear.

Remember the inner mind does not work with logic. If it did then patterns formed in childhood and at times of trauma would no longer affect us as we mature. The inner mind may be telling us something that no amount of conscious guess-work could understand. If we talk to it using its own 'language' then we are sure of understanding without confusion, but only if we talk using its version of the world, not ours.

Everyone can symbolise better under hypnosis. Recognition is based on energy patterns, just as all sensory recognition is, and we can use our imagination to both access and change those patterns momentarily or permanently.

How we use this in the hypnosis session is simplicity itself. Say I wish to deal with a fear or phobia. I reduce the sensory input and ask their mind for a symbol for that fear. It may well happen that the symbol makes them feel some, if not all, of the emotions attached to the symbol. It isn't always the case and it doesn't matter if they do or don't.

To change the issue and its attached emotional patterns is then very simple, change the symbol. You can do this any way you like. My preferred method is to put it in their hands and get them to physically change it. I will often ask them to get the symbol for what they want to achieve and get them to mould the two together. I then take them to their **perfect place** which we talk about in the next chapter and have them put it in a place of honour. And that is that.

Quick, simple and effective.

Perfect Places

I don't know who invented this metaphor but I've been using it along with direct suggestion for ever. I just like it. And it fits in with symbolism like a dream and that's great because the dream world is after all where we work.

I have been told that the following is very reminiscent of the work that Dreamweavers like Imhotep in ancient Egypt did. It certainly reminds me of the sort of thing reported by American Indians when visiting the spirit plane. And by Aborigines when they go walkabout.

What we do is get the hypnotee to create their place, their perfect place. This can be anywhere, and any time in the universe. This is the place where they can feel calm, tranquil, safe, and secure. The temperature is perfect, the lighting is just right; everything about this place is comfortable. "Nothing can enter or leave this place apart from you and the sound of my voice".

Notice how this is worded to be ambiguous and not to lead. Their perfect place should come from them, not you.

This is a wonderful tool.

We can use this place to increase recall and accelerate learning. Tell them to create a unique receptacle into which they can put anything special they need to remember. They can create a different receptacle for every occasion.

This is the most amazing memory aid I've ever seen. I suspect that it works simply because we never deliberately put anything away we need to remember in our heads. Using this metaphor though we create a filing system and instead of our mind rushing around trying to find where it put something it just goes straight to the appropriate place. This works with anything you want to anchor not just facts and stuff. Even emotions can be stored and retrieved.

A friend once said to me that it was a shame you couldn't bottle joy. Using the perfect place, your symbol for joy, and a handy receptacle, you can bottle the emotion, at least in your internal reality. And lets face it, that's where you really live. Just create the place, the receptacle and fill it, and you can retrieve those feeling whenever you need them.

As with hypnotic symbolism the trick for the hypnotist is don't impose what your idea of a perfect place is. Never tell them what this could be or should look like.

Magic Metaphor

Using metaphor is the most creative way of engaging the hypnotic process for change. And it can be argued that all we ever do is work with metaphors because reality is subjective anyway. I use metaphor of course with symbolism, but it isn't my number one way of working. But it could just be that you find it fits you better than direct suggestion. So I've included it for you, just in case.

Metaphor in hypnosis isn't just using a phrase to represent something else; it's much more like telling a story. That is telling a story with a moral or result which empowers the needed change in your people.

Vince Montgomery of Swindon, one of the best naturals at creative metaphors I've ever had the pleasure to teach on a course, used the metaphor of a river flow being interrupted by rocks when asked to help with a stammer.

In conversation before the hypnosis Vince discovered the guy had a passion for fly fishing and used this to easily fire the guy's anchors of feeling good by 'placing' him in the water.

Vince then suggested that some rocks were blocking the flow of the water and that the water was just like words.

The guy then threw the rocks away to allow the river of words to flow more easily. The guy was actually miming throwing the rocks out, really struggling with one or two. At the end of the process the guy could speak clearly and with no stammer.

It should by now be obvious that nearly everything we do is actually metaphor. The perfect place is metaphor. Receptacles are metaphors for our brain.

Relaxation is a metaphor, and so is the induced sleep that most people think of when they think of hypnosis.

So a metaphor is a story or imagined situation which represents the hypnotees' inner reality. Sounds a bit like symbolism doesn't it? Except that in this case the metaphor comes from the hypnotist.

This is probably the easiest way to work with kids. Unlike with adults, where the metaphor has to be delivered around the conscious, even a kid's immature conscious mind is usually up for a story.

The trick with these small people is to make the story recognisable.

Find out what the child's favourite TV show, play station game or even on the odd occasion, what their best book is.

Watch, play, or read this to get the right feel for it and use a metaphoric situation with all their favourite characters and heroes in it. Use a situation where the required change can be aided and anchors set up.

On one of our classes Vitalijs, a delegate from Latvia, got stumped on metaphor because of the cultural differences. But he and his hypnotee had been talking about their shared liking for music so Vitalijs started speaking the words of a song he knew to his hypnotee. The thing worked like a charm as it appealed massively to the recipient's emotive mind under hypnosis and 'Up where we belong', got rid of an issue with heights wonderfully well.

We are surrounded by metaphor. For growth we could use a tree; an eradication of the taught feelings of stress can be an elastic band; and the brothers Grimm and Disney have given us a whole library of metaphorical stories, each with their own very handy moral and metaphor.

To decide which metaphor best fits your clients discover their passion and use that.

The following was posted to our Yahoo discussion group on the Internet by a fellow of the Academy, Cat Milton.

"Quite simply, I find out what passions my clients have.

One 54yr old woman (Auto-immune system problems) had a passion for Patrick Stewart (Star Trek!!).

Under hypnosis I took her through the visualisation of Patrick Stewart going in and commanding her immune system back to good health and balance.

I linked the session to a favourite piece of her music and each time she went to sleep at night listening to the music with the direction that her body would get better and better.

Perhaps not surprisingly, when she left hospital one of the first things she did was see Patrick Stewart at some play in London! *chuckle*. Another client had a passion for painting sea creatures - fish, shells etc.

She had a particular love of sea horses so under hypnosis we built her an army of sea horses to course thru' her body, fixing it.

I saw her once a week for 12 weeks and, after 9 years of a crippling disease, she has returned to full time work - and has a lovely set of sea horse paintings to mark each week of her recovery
:-) " Cat

Metaphor is all around us, from Santa to Willy Wonka, and is an elegant and useful way to deliver suggestion.

Easy, Long-term Issue Resolution

One of the hardest things for hypnotherapists and psychologists to do is to let go of their own perspective, especially that of time.

The problem is that we always look at how big or small we feel we are from where we are on our perceived timeline. And quite naturally we look at other people in the same way. It is human nature to see everything above us on the timeline as less significant, and everything below us as more important.

Socially, we tend to give respect to people older than us based on the amount of time that they have hung around, often regardless of whether they've done anything particularly respect-provoking with their lives. Try as hard as we might, adults really do look down on children, and not just physically. I know we really do make the effort to treat them as little people, which in my opinion is totally the inappropriate thing to do, but deep inside we know that they have a lot to learn and in our time sphere they are easy to deal with because they know little and their timeline isn't as long or important as ours. They haven't been around enough.

We tend to apply this thinking to our behaviour with what we see as issues, thinking that because something has been around for a long time then it must be more complex, or difficult to get rid of. We give it gravitas and respect, regardless of whether it's done anything for us. So if something's been around for a long time it's only logical to assume it's going to take a long time to get rid of it.

This isn't my experience.

In my thinking old doesn't mean complicated.

I think to get the right perspective on how long or how hard an issue is to resolve you have to consider how long it took to get it in the first place. A behaviour doesn't grow, for that matter neither does a belief. In fact our emotional patterns are all formed in an instant.

I know it might be hard to grasp this. Mainly because you were taught at school by repetition. So the pattern you have for learning is one of repetition. And that pattern is wrong. I think that when you learn something you learn it in the moment when your mind is dominant. It's at that time when you are open to suggestion and if that's accepted then the pattern is built.

Of course in schools where the teachers are not trained hypnotists, or even know that's what's happening, we must use repetition. Then sooner or later we are going to hit some of the children at a time when they will accept the patterns we are giving them. Of course that also means that if we don't excite them or get them to feel really emotive about the subject, get them passionate and get them hypnotised, then no amount of repetition will teach them anything, except of course to be bored.

Think about this yourself. What did you find hardest to learn at school? Was it the subjects you were really passionate and emotive about or the stuff you felt was mundane? We actually remember that stuff better as well.

I remember at the age of eight or nine we were taught parrot fashion to sing the carol 'All through the night' in Welsh and guess what, although I knew every syllable then, I can't recall a single word now. But ask me to sing 'Love me do' by the Beatles and I'll happily murder that from start to finish.

The carol took weeks to learn, the lyrics of the pop song only took one or two plays. The fact is the carol was hard work, and the Beatles song was "Fab".

Learning that song took longer than a phobia takes to put into place and maybe that's why the phobia has such strength, because it doesn't come with any doubts if we can do it.

Unusually my experience validates psychotherapeutic theory that there is a **trigger event** for all behaviour, and it is this trigger event that becomes the suggestion. Accepted, this then becomes the internal reality which becomes the pattern for behaviour and belief.

I remember one of my brothers telling me that there was a wardrobe monster living at the bottom of my mother's wardrobe. From that moment on for years I wouldn't enter my mother's bedroom if the wardrobe door was open.

That particular suggestion didn't need any compounding (that is repetition proving the reality and giving it strength) or longevity. I was scared from that moment until a time that reality was replaced by something stronger in the form of a new wardrobe and a sledge hammer.

Truth is I still feel slightly uncomfortable with an open door in a bedroom. Maybe I should see a hypnotist?

The established thought is this, it can be harder to get rid of a condition that has been around for a long time and that behaviours grow in strength through time. This being the case then it will take a commensurate amount of time to rid the client of their affliction. So the equation amounts to "duration of behaviour = amount of difficulty in eradication = time of the eradication". So a thirty year issue will take quite a few sessions and a deal of time to get rid of.

However my opinion is that the equation we should be using as hypnotists is:

length of trigger event = time of the eradication.

If a phobia takes an instant to install then, because we are using the same process, it should only take an instant to remove. The same can be said of all emotional conditions. And it's easier to work that way. As I say in masterclasses old doesn't mean hard.

For that reason I see no correlation between the amount of time an issue has been in place and the difficulty of removing it. If you adopt this view you will find that you approach even the most complex and tricky conditions with much more confidence. This will reflect in both the efficacy of your technique and in the rapidity of the success you will have with your client.

The other thing to consider about time is that for the mind it doesn't exist. That's why we see no sense of how much time passes in moments of trauma, emotional excess or sleep or hypnosis. The brain uses time but the inner reality is that there is only now. So for the mind a long term problem started now, just in a different now.

You can work at the speed of the only thing that exceeds the speed of light, and that my friend is the speed of thought. Why work any slower?

Play Hypnosis

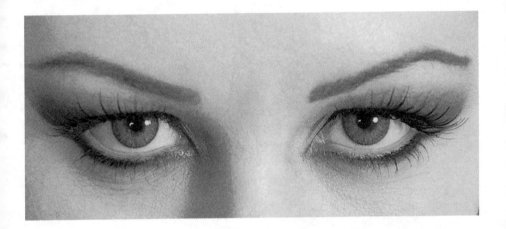

An illuminating and amusing diversion from the cares and pressures of everyday life hypnosis can be a wonderful toy to explore a fascinating, moving and wonderfully creative reality.

I know this might make some therapists shake in their boots as they feel insecure enough that any non-serious use of hypnosis would be seen as undermining their validity. Personally I've never felt this to be the case. In fact in my experience having fun and exploring have always gone a long way to increasing both my reputation and my client base.

Now, we are not talking about stage hypnosis here, as the point is not to amuse an audience. Rather it is the job of the hypnotist to demonstrate to the hypnotees themselves the amazing and wondrous world of the alternative reality we can all create and to amuse and amaze the ourselves.

It's like day dreaming on steroids and could be a valuable service for the hypnotist to offer clients who want to just experience and who have no need for healing, therapy or trickcyclery.

Now before my internal picture of a hypnotherapist / psychotherapist loading a shotgun becomes reality let me just say that escapism from what is for some a mundane life is the norm with the average human being. There is absolutely nothing wrong in such diversion.

In fact play is a healthy way of controlling stress and of course it goes without saying that children learn more in their first five or six years of life at play than they ever do after starting 'serious' school and developing a work ethic and losing the play ethic.

It is being able to create our own inner reality and to use imagination to occupy some of our daily experience that sets us apart from other living entities and although hypnosis is able to be used .

Maybe that's what mind was made to do. Play and enjoy and experience this totally amazing place we call a universe.

We daydream, we play games on a computer, we watch television and films and of course we read books. We also write books and create something of beauty from totally inert and lifeless substances. If we are not inventing our own reality we'll usually experience someone else's.

There is absolutely nothing whatsoever at all wrong with escapism unless the chosen method is detrimental to the person using it in a significant way as in the case of watching re-runs of Friends. I am of course referring to the use of drugs. Not just the big 'illegal' drugs either.

Alcohol, tobacco, coffee and all sorts of food substances are used to escape or alleviate the effects of 'reality'. Even then this is a choice thing and as such is entirely down to the individual providing it doesn't harm anyone else, which sadly all of the above tend to do.

Whether this is inappropriate or not is of course entirely subjective, but let's just suppose for a moment that most of the things people bring to us hypnotists asking for their eradication from their lives are actually inappropriate. After all, this book is for the hypnotist and even though you must never impose your reality on others, you have to take a stand somewhere. The idea of a hypnotist who sits on the fence makes me shudder.

That aside let's just take a quick look at the sort of thing you could offer people to allow them to enjoy the capability of the hypnotic state and to empower and increase their capacity to enjoy both the sensual and imaginary.

A drug free 'High'

A standard with a lot of UK stage hypnotists is to suggest that the volunteer is smoking a substance which normally would cause them a great deal of trouble if there was a handy policeman patrolling. That is, smoking marijuana or pot. The interesting thing is that when I have done this in the past the incumbents react in a very similar manner to the suggestion as they would to smoking the plant itself. And I have been told that the experienced effect is exactly the same. Although we are talking the experience here because, obviously, no substance enters the body.

Now, if you remember, the hypnotee has to be able to imagine what the suggested reality would be like. And if you experiment with this and know what you're looking for you can certainly tell those who have from those who haven't, although when instructed to remember the event they all report the same strangely mixed feeling of euphoria and tranquillity that apparently such substances can apparently create. Personally it just makes me puke, however an imagined high doesn't paint the walls in a lovely shade of vomit.

I'll let your mind play with the potential for some interesting experiments you may be able to set up with this one. The benefits of experiencing the desired emotional effects whilst avoiding the undesired physical and addictive aspects should be obvious.

Interestingly enough a lot of people in the past have used such material to increase their creativity, to increase the capability of stepping aside from their normal reality. It's a fact that the huge amount of creative thinking and inventiveness of the human race has happened during such substance supported play and diversion.

There are many deliciously enjoyable experiences which can benefit by the heightened emotional response of both the mind and the brain. A visit to the local theme park will demonstrate quite easily that fear, definitely our strongest emotion; can be as enjoyable as it is destructive. We even go out of our way to increase its effects. Although told quite clearly to **'Keep hands inside'** we don't, do we?

At the biggest rides how many of us have spent boring time in the line regaling everyone with stories of the time it broke and maimed several thousand people and squished a cat. This is suggestive metaphor at its best.

Hypnosis can be used to experience this whole thing without the waiting and with no harm to any cats. The question is should you charge for Play or Fun hypnosis?

Why not?

The thing is that not everyone is ill, sick or demented and I see no reason why hypnosis should be used only to repair and remedy when it can be used for so much more.

As a hypnotist, rather than as a hypnotherapist, it's interesting to note that there is a lucrative and fascinating market which has been left largely unexplored in commercial terms. The number one form of 'play' enjoyed by adults in the vast majority of countries and cultures, certainly western ones, is that of exploring their sexuality.

There is absolutely no doubt that hypnotic states can increase the physical sensuality and lengthen both the experience and affect of this most enjoyable pastime.

Just consider that the industry that has grown up around adult sexual play and alternative life styles is worth billions every year. And that isn't just because there are lots of perverts but because there are billions of people who just like sex. Why shouldn't hypnosis be offered to those who just enjoy the feelings of heightened emotion and physical sensuality it offers?

There is no doubt in my mind that enjoyment and entertainment, escapism and play are quite possibly more therapeutic and certainly more preventative than any issue based clinical approach.

For that reason the play element of hypnotic suggestion should be used more. All you have to do is create the state, implant anchors for whatever result you wish, and play.

Also by Jonathan Chase

DEEPER AND DEEPER

the secrets of stage hypnosis

Jonathan Chase's best selling book on modern stage hypnosis is now used world wide as a definitive reference on the subject of fast and funny entertainment hypnosis and by hypnotherapists as a guide to fast inductions and powerful suggestions. Covering Showmanship, Suggestion, Safety, the "Dream Pilot" tells it all in this complete instruction. Note: this book is entirely free when you enrol on the Stage Hypnosis Masterclass.

"A wonderful new book by England's hypnotist, Jonathan Chase, is a great way to start performing the art of Stage Hypnosis."

Bryan Dean - MagicTalk

"Deeper and Deeper is very matter of fact. It is written with great weight and authority because it is the distillation of decades of real life experience, devoid of speculation or theory."

Barry Thain – Clinical Hypnotist

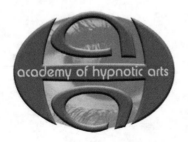

STAGE HYPNOSIS MASTERCLASS

The secrets of stage hypnosis revealed in this 2 disc comprehensive DVD

As in his book Deeper and Deeper the secrets of stage hypnosis, and in the Live School of Stage Hypnosis Masterclasses, the attention to safety, care and respect for the volunteers is paramount in the underlying philosophy of Jonathan Chase.

In this unique training presentation you are taken from live masterclass footage, to the preparations for a show in front of an invited audience of hypnotists and guests, in a specially edited version of that show with Jon's comments revealing the thought process and 'secret stuff' going on constantly in the background.

"I've found it really useful and have used several ideas from it."
Paul Dawkins

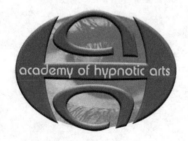

BY JONATHAN CHASE

ALSO AVAILABLE FROM
ACADEMY OF HYPNOTIC ARTS LTD

Deeper and Deeper the secrets of stage hypnosis £14.95

Stage Hypnosis Masterclass 2 set DVD £55

Please send cheque/ (sterling and US dollar only) credit or debit card.

Expiry Date:_____

Signature _____

Please allow £2.50 for post and packing in UK.

Overseas customers please allow £3.50 for post and packing.

ALL ORDERS TO:
Academy of Hypnotic Arts Ltd.
PO Box 82
Dawlish, Devon. EX7 0WP

NAME: _____

ADDRESS: _____

_____

_____

_____

EMAIL: _____

PHONE: _____

☐ Please tick box if you do not wish
to receive further information.

Please allow 28 days for delivery.

Prices and availability subject to change without notice.